For Dr... and.
Affectionate))
Isadore Seeman
Seen

THE TWENTIETH CENTURY THROUGH MY EYES

BY
ISADORE SEEMAN

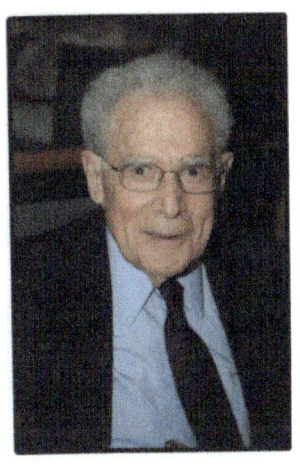

Summit Crossroads Press
First Person History Series
Columbia, Md

Published in the United States of America by
    Summit Crossroads Press
    Columbia, Maryland
    E-mail Address: sumcross@aol.com

The author may be reached by e-mail at samseeman1@gmail.com

ISBN: 978-0-9614519-3-6

Library of Congress Control No. 2015960945

PREFACE

Summing up a life, a full lifetime, demands more than the enumeration of events and dates, the recitation of the plusses and minuses. Life is an emotional journey. Until you understand the passions that drive the experience forward, hear the laughter and envision the tears, you cannot appreciate the person, you do not share the enterprise. I hope this tome reveals who I was and what my life has meant, against the background of the times in which I lived.

It is the tale of the son of immigrants, in a family limited by poverty until the children attained advanced education and moved on. I, the fourth of five children, chose a career in public health and community organization after an experience with tuberculosis.

My three brothers each achieved a Ph.D and all served as professors in universities. My sister, the only girl in the family, suffered a handicapping illness in childhood, but grew up to serve in nursing, to marry, and raise two successful children. I had the great opportunity to play a leadership role for 18 years in advancing health and welfare services in the National Capital Area; a more rewarding experience is hard to imagine.

Now, at 99, I look back on almost a century, a volatile century that endured eight wars, the development and use of the atomic bomb, vast social changes, and great technological advances. Through this narrative and through my poetry I have sought to understand and convey meaning out of my relationships and my life. You can judge the result.

THE BEGINNING IN BALTIMORE
1916

I grew up in Baltimore, Maryland, where I was born on August 15, completed my early education, was married, had our first child, and lived until I was 33 years old. In the early years, from birth to graduation from high school, I lived in a family that was financially poor, emotionally strained, under tension between parents at odds with each other, and on the move every few years, occupying ten different houses in ten different neighborhoods, largely because my father was unable to earn enough income to support seven people.

Our parents were almost constantly disagreeing, angry at each other, not communicating. Our mother was the strong parent, very caring, nurturing her children, advising and guiding, and perhaps above all, determined that her children receive a good education. Our father was immature, childlike, unable to feel or show affection to his wife or his children, and an overbearing disciplinarian.

When I was born, Woodrow Wilson was president of the U.S. He served from March 1913 to March 1921.

After graduation I enjoyed two exciting and glorious years in a community theatre, acting, and learning and practicing backstage scenic and lighting techniques. Then reality took over, and circumstances forced me to spend three years at Towson State Teachers College, following the footsteps of my three brothers. Graduating in 1938 with a teaching certificate but no academic degree, I started to contribute to the family finances as did my three brothers by teaching in the Baltimore City public schools. Imagine all four Seeman brothers now teachers, all in the city school system. We were close in all things, on dates, all four sitting in the second balcony of the downtown theatre, meeting at the new central public library downtown, and in "family councils."

After two years teaching, an illness changed my life. I discovered that I had tuberculosis, and spent 14 months lying flat on my back on an open porch in a sanatorium outside of Baltimore, summer and winter, to rest my lungs and allow them to destroy the tubercle bacillus. With unlimited time to think and plan, I decided that no one needed to get tuberculosis; it was a contagion that was preventable. I was determined to make a career of public health.

World War I

Eight months after I was born, the Congress of the United States declared war on Germany, and we were engaged in World War I. The war began in July 1914 shortly after the assassination of Archduke Franz Ferdinand, heir to the Austrian throne, by a Yugoslav nationalist. More fundamentally, the war grew out of the imperialist policies of the great powers of Europe. The German Empire, the Austro-Hungarian Empire, the Ottoman Empire, the Russian Empire, and the empires of Britain, France, and Italy clashed, and their colonies became involved. The Allies opposed the Central Powers. In all, 70 million military personnel participated, and nine million combatants were killed.

Austro-Hungary invaded Serbia, and Germany invaded Belgium, Luxembourg, and France. Russia advanced against Austro-Hungary, then was beaten back by Germany. The Ottoman Empire joined in 1914, Italy and Bulgaria in 1915, and Romania in 1916. In 1917 the Russian Empire collapsed and after the October revolution, Russia left the war.

President Woodrow Wilson kept the United States out of the war, until seven U.S. merchant ships were sunk by German submarines. Congress declared war in April 1917. Congress passed the

Selective Service Act, and 2.8 million men were drafted. The Allies were successful, and Germany agreed to a cease fire on November 11, 1918. The Treaty of Versailles was signed, and the map of Central Europe was redrawn. The League of Nations was formed in an effort to avert future wars.

After I started teaching, aware that I would need a degree to advance in any profession, I took evening classes at Johns Hopkins University. There I met the person who would become my wife. She, too, was seeking education, to advance from a secretarial career. We "dated" until I was hospitalized, and she visited me regularly at the sanatorium. After I was discharged and found a new position, earning the then-great sum of $2,400 a year, we married. Details of our early years come later.

I was born at 1920 Fleet Street in Baltimore City. For most people, that statement would mean that my parents lived at that address when they brought me home from the hospital. In my case, it was a different experience. My parents' culture and poverty—they could surely not afford a physician and a stay in a hospital—produced a different event.

I was born at home; my mother was delivered by a midwife, with no physician in attendance. I can vouch for the validity of this event—my birth certificate. Some 28 years later I served as director of the Bureau of Vital Records of the Baltimore City Health Department where all records of births and deaths in the city are filed. I looked up my birth record and found the entry: Isador (later changed to Isadore) Seeman, born August 15, 1916, mother's maiden name Sophie Kostman, age 25, birthplace Austria, and father Morris Seeman, age 29, birthplace Austria, occupation shoemaker. The midwife was Mary Mrozinski. The birth occurred at 1920 Fleet Street at 9 a.m. Thus it began; my entry into the world.

Baltimore is a very old city, settled in 1729 as a seaport. It served for a brief few months in 1776 as the capital of the country when Philadelphia had to be evacuated for safety. By 1800 it was the third largest city in the U.S. In 1920, a few years after I was born, its population of 733,826 made it the sixth largest city in the country. It was a thriving seaport, shipbuilding and steelmaking city, with a rich culture and immigrants from many countries: Poles, Germans, Italians, and Jews, living in distinct neighborhoods. It is unique in that it is an independent city,

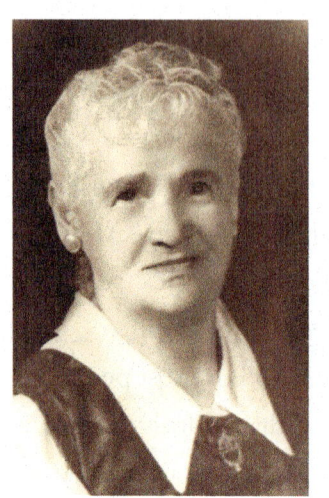

My mother.

not located in any county. Its location on the Patapsco River makes it a part of the Chesapeake Bay.

My mother was born in Stryj on January 4, 1891. Stryj was located sometimes in Austria, sometimes in Poland, and perhaps in the Ukraine, as borders changed in those years. My father was born in a small town near Stryj. My birth certificate states that he was born in 1887, but another estimate is that he was born on March 15, 1886.

My mother wrote a brief autobiography in later years, and more of that later, but she does describe the courtship. My father was eager to marry her and pursued her, but she initially declined. He later was drafted into the Austrian army, and when he returned, he resumed the courtship. At this point she succumbed and agreed, although her reluctance was clear. My father apprenticed as a shoemaker and actually made shoes in Europe. My mother was apprenticed to a dressmaker and was skilled at this throughout her life.

My father came to America in 1912, seeking a better life than the Shtetl (small town) in Austria offered a Jewish family. He left behind his wife and two children, Will and Gussie. As I grew curious about our genealogy in later years, and also interested my son David in this endeavor, he found a copy of the ship's manifest that included my father's name: it was the S.S. Brandenburg, sailing from Bremen and arriving in America.

At that time Baltimore was an alternative entry port to the United States instead of Ellis Island in New York. He had decided to leave Europe, get established in America, and then bring his wife and two children to join him. My mother came in 1914 on the S.S. Armenia with two babies; Will, age 2, and Gussie, age 11/12. (That's what the manifest shows.) She often said she came on the last ship to arrive before World War I.

I have limited memories of my early childhood. As happens fre-

The five children. Left to right: Jules, Mef, Izz., Gussie, Will.

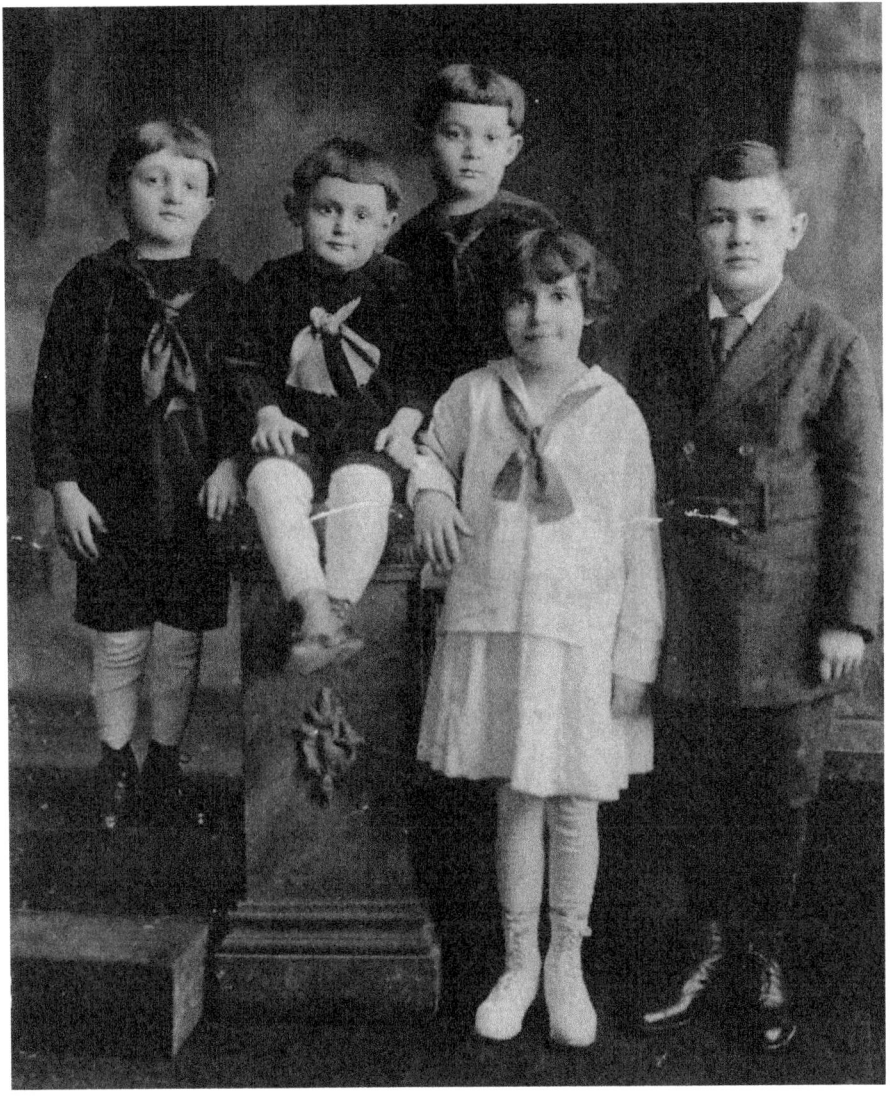

quently, it is difficult to separate original memories from recalls at family gatherings where earlier experiences are recounted.

I entered a family that consisted of my father Morris, my mother Sophia, my oldest brother Will (William), then age four, my sister Gussie (Augusta), then age 3; and my brother Jules (Julius), age one and one-half, the first of the children born in the U.S. The last of the family entered 18 months after I was born--Mef (Melvin). We five children were the clan. A little arithmetic will reveal that all five of us were born just about 18 months apart; that speaks to my father's sexual proclivity, and the absence of birth control.

My parents' life in Europe and entry to the United States is clouded in an untold history. That generation spoke little of their life in Europe or their trip to America, and the children all too seldom inquired.

There is a fascinating sidelight on our family name, emanating from a little-known custom in Europe. My father was the son of Esther Seeman who married Harry Wolfe Hirschman; hence my father's name was Morris Hirschman. My father was drafted into the Austrian army, and when he reported for duty he was asked to produce identity papers. Among the records requested was his parents' marriage certificate. My father had none. His parents were married by a rabbi and never by a civilian authority, hence no civil marriage record existed. Under Austrian law, absent a marriage record, he was his mother's child, and his father was not recognized. My mother's maiden name was Esther Seeman. Thus the authorities recorded him as Morris Seeman, a child only of his mother. That name stuck with him, and we are now Seeman, not Hirschman.

The house where I was born was a storefront with rooms in the rear and on the second floor. The store is where my father repaired shoes. In Europe he had been a shoemaker—literally; he made shoes. I do remember the machines he used to smooth the leather soles and rubber heels; they fascinated a child. I can see him cutting the leather for a new sole, using a special knife with a perpendicular edge to guide the cut. I re-

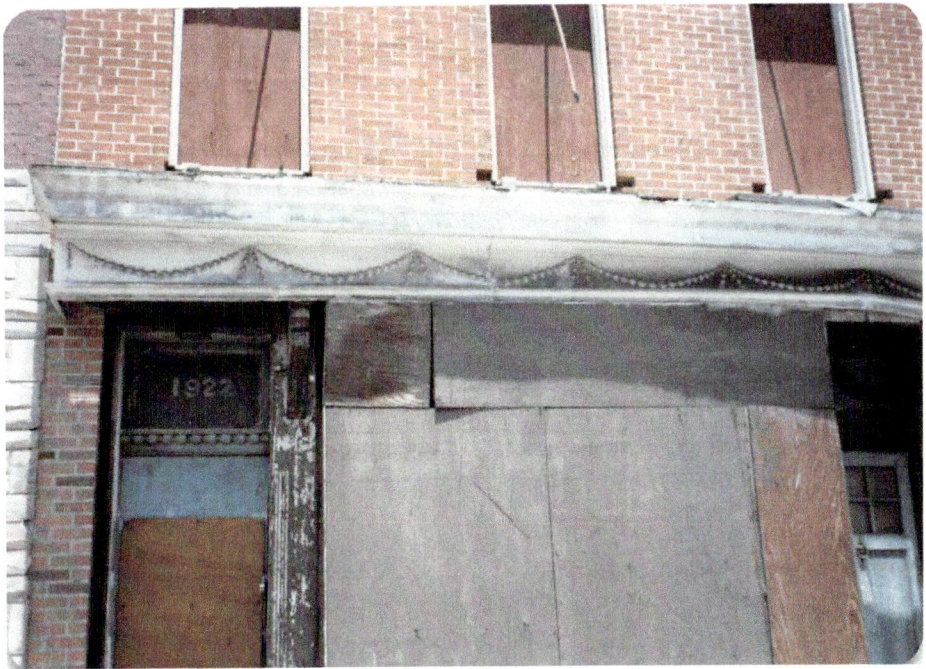

1920 Fleet Street, the house where I was born.

member, too, how he pounded the small nails into the edges of the soles, placed on a special metal device shaped like a shoe. For efficiency, he put several small nails into his mouth and extracted them one by one as he hammered the soles. I can also see (and smell) the glue he used to help hold the soles in place, and awe at the machines he used.

I have been back to that neighborhood a number of times; some just for remembrance, once to show my wife; once to show my nephew Paul from California. Obviously some memories of the neighborhood are original and some are from the later visits. The most remarkable recollection is the fact that a railroad line for freight ran on Fleet Street, directly in front of our house. I do not recall seeing the trains run there in my childhood, but a later memory probably reflects what happened there. When I was 12 or 13 years old, I delivered the *Baltimore Sun* every morning about 3 a.m. on a route in south Baltimore. A freight train ran on one of the streets on my route. I can see a man preceding the train, riding on a white horse, and warning traffic at the cross streets of the train's approach.

What happened in 1916, my birth year
*The battle of Verdon, and the battle of the Somme
occurred in World War I.
There was an anti-British rebellion in Ireland, the Easter Rising.
Margaret Sanger opened the first birth control clinic in the U.S.,
in Brooklyn, N.Y.
The U.S. National Park Service was created.
Charlie Chaplin signed a movie contract for the
high price of $10,000 a week.
Albert Einstein completed his general theory of relativity.*

Obviously I do not remember these events; I looked them up for this biography.

We did not have a bathtub, and certainly not a shower, in the house. I remember walking with my father to the public baths several blocks from our house every Sunday morning to get our weekly shower.

I can picture the school where I attended. Though I was not aware of it, I was enrolled in kindergarten a year ahead of the established date for admission. My mother's passionate devotion to the education of her children evidenced itself that early by enrolling each of her children a year before the established age. I recall that when I was in junior high school the teacher was checking the age of each child. When she came to me, she challenged my report of my age, since the school record was a year off.

Will as the oldest son was just learning English, since my parents spoke only Yiddish to each other and were themselves just learning English. Will started school a year ahead of the established time, speaking little English. We lived in a predominately Polish neighborhood, where anti-Semitism was common. Will often came home chased and beaten by Polish kids who taunted him. My father could speak Polish. (I remember one of the curse words he sometimes used, after an annoying customer left—"Shakref Schwinia"—Damned swine.)

Perhaps the most often cited recollection of "the boys" in our childhood is of the changes in "pairing" among us. One day, Will and Jules as the two oldest were heading off on some adventure and did not wish Mef and me, the two youngest, to tag along. So I picture Mef and me sitting on the step in front of our house being told to stay behind, and our reward would be that when they returned, they would bring us a pony. I'm still looking for that pony.

We had a dog named Tim when we were children. There was also a policeman on the beat with whom we got acquainted, also named Tim. The dog unfortunately chased cars as they drove along Fleet Street, and he was killed in one of these chases.

I was visiting in a neighbor's house one day, and their dog apparently felt I was a threat to him. He bit me on the cheek; the scar is still visible.

One of my father's cousins, Abe Seaman, had a used furniture store a few blocks from our house, and we kids visited there. For reasons we do not understand, he spelled his name Seaman. There was another of my father's cousins, Ellis, who also had a used furniture store, this one in Highlandtown. He, too, spelled his name Seaman.

My mother was religious and kept kosher. My father went along, though he was less observant. We attended an orthodox "shul" (synagogue) on Bond Street. One of my father's uncles, Koppel Seaman, also lived on Bond Street. Each Sunday the family would gather there, and the men played poker I remember standing at my father's shoulder watching the game. At times when the game was held in our house, my mother would collect a nickel from every pot to pay for the food that was served at the poker games—deli sandwiches.

There were children our ages among the cousins. My father had two sisters who came to America; Sophie who married Ben Greenberg, a barber, and had two daughters, Annie and Minnie. The second sister, Pauline, lived in East Orange, New Jersey. She married Louis Cohen, a tailor, and had three children, Will, Motie, and Esther. I do recall one younger child, a son of Abe's, who was being toilet trained and had an accident in his father's store. Abe shouted at him; it was so impressive that I remember the Yiddish words, "Farfalte pisher, lig und fahl dou" (disgraceful pisser, lie and fall here).

Years later when I visited the neighborhood, our store front had been removed and replaced by an ordinary residence. A vague recollection is about the next door—1922 Fleet Street. We may have owned or used this other house at some point.

What was the atmosphere in the family? It can best be understood from an autobiography my mother wrote for a short time in 1963, at age 72, that is very revealing and very moving. She lived an unhappy life with her husband. She wrote the first page in Yiddish. We had it translated.

She wrote:
"Dear White Paper,

I can pour out to you my pain from my bitter heart. You will not be able to tell my hurt; it will remain only for me and you. It is hard to live in one house with a person who doesn't understand you, has no feeling for human beings, and no sensitivity, and will not try to understand the worth of a partnership. He does things on the spur of the moment without thinking and without discussing it. And you cannot help yourself. You talk to yourself and it hurts very bitterly." Some other excerpts: "I would like very much to be able to put down on paper my story; I believe it could make interesting reading and maybe someone could learn what not to do in order to make life more pleasant." And this: "Oh, God, please help me, show me the way to a little happiness. It is so little that I ask for, and I think I'm satisfied with so little, but there is no understanding, no cooperation. I'm suffering; I'm miserable but in order not to shame myself and the children I have to go on with my life as it is."

This is the background in which I grew up. In spite of my mother's hope and wish to keep her anguish from the children, it came through.

Throughout our lifetime, my parents had innumerable disagreements. My father was hard to live with. He never achieved maturity—always self-absorbed, very opinionated, disrespectful of other's views, childlike in many ways. He worked at shoe repair and selling new shoes, but never made a good living. We were poor throughout our growing-up years. We called our father Pop. My mother supplemented our family income by taking in foster children, sometimes as many as three. (I remember once we had twins living with us.) My mother was the strong parent, very intelligent, very determined to protect the family, to assure a good education for her children. As Will was finishing high school, my father said he should find a job and go to work. My mother put her foot down firmly; her sons were going to get more education, one way or another. Will got an after-school job that brought some money into the house.

Our house was heated by coal kept in the cellar to stoke the furnace. My father would often go down to the cellar and brood when he had a fight with my mother. I have a vivid recollection of Will crawling under the kitchen table to get away from my father who was chasing him with a strap (belt) in his hand. My father called my mother "Zeesel" which is Yiddish for sweet. Considering their relationship, it was the most inappropriate name possible.

MOVING—TEN TIMES

My father decided that he was not doing sufficient business on Fleet Street. He decided to move to another neighborhood. We moved to 2251 E. Biddle Street, again with a store front and living area behind and upstairs. This was a nicer house in a nicer neighborhood. The elementary school was directly across the street. I was in third grade when we moved, and my adjustment at the new school was difficult, so I failed the third grade. I remember the embarrassed and mortifying feeling on being told to move to the front desk in the room because I was going to remain in the same grade. (I later skipped one grade, so I compensated for the failure.)

What happened in 1917?
The U.S. entered World War I.
The Russian revolution began. Czar Nicholas II abdicated.
The Balfour declaration was proclaimed expressing British support for a
Jewish national home in Palestine.
The worldwide influenza epidemic started; by 1920
20 million people died.
Between 10,000 and 15,000 blacks walked silently down Fifth Avenue
in New York to protest racial discrimination.

After attending public school each day, we went to "cheder" (Hebrew School) at the Baltimore Talmud Torah. (Will started his Hebrew education at a different "Cheder" with a teacher who cracked their knuckles with a ruler when they did poorly.) To encourage us to go when we protested, my mother gave us each a few pennies a day, and we regularly bought a pickle and a pretzel on the way. I remember not liking the idea of going, but once I got there it was not too bad. We studied Hebrew, some Jewish history, but in all a pretty dull experience. I remember one lesson that made me proud: the assignment was to make a list of Hebrew nouns in which the male and female were completely different words. (Most Hebrew female nouns are the male with only a different ending.) I observed that the words for male and female fell into the category the teacher wanted—they are Zachar (male) and Nekevah (female), completely different words for the different genders.

One incident in our experience on Biddle Street impressed me. A cowboy in a circus that had come to town came to the store to have my father repair his cowboy boots. He gave us passes to see the circus.

We had a fence in the yard at the back of the house. I remember climbing over the fence one day in a game we were playing. There was a nail in the fence, and I caught my hand on the nail. The stitches in my hand are still visible.

It was during our stay on Biddle Street that my father bought his first car; a used Hupmobile. He drove the family one Sunday as far as the towns in southern Pennsylvania. I recall that he remarked about all of the "foreign" license plates when he observed the Pennsylvania tags.

What happened in 1918?
The second battle of the Marne took place.
The former Czar of Russia was executed.
The German Kaiser, Wilhelm II, abdicated.
The influenza pandemic raged.
World War I ended with an armistice signed at 11 a.m.
on the 11th day of the 11th month.

There was a small neighborhood park about two blocks from our house. We often went there to play—shooting marbles, playing mumbley peg with a pen knife, playing caddie (hitting a small stick with its ends cut to a point and hitting it with a larger stick), and certainly running games like Home Sheep Run.

Will had a close friend named Sander Solomon, whose father owned a hardware store. Occasionally we joined them in games. I had a friend named Meyer Stollar. About a block away was a Jewish family named Bugatch, who owned a tailor shop. They bought a radio when such devices were rare. We kids joined my father there to listen to prize fights. One incident in childhood that I recall vividly: I took Mef to see a movie I was very interested in—a historical film. During the movie Mef felt ill, and I had to take him home. I was very disappointed to leave the movie.

The four boys were close to each other in those early years. Gussie was not only the one sister; in childhood she developed an illness that affected her brain—probably meningitis or encephalitis. She was placed in special homes for many years, so she was not part of the close family during that period. She never regained normalcy, but was able to cope. In later years she studied nursing and worked as a nurse. She married quite late, and her husband was difficult to live with. She made every effort to control her family and assure a good education for her children, struggling against the opposition of her husband to paying for college for their son. Both children, Esther and Harvey, grew to attain very successful careers.

One characteristic of my childhood, which continued throughout my life, was observed by my father when he said, "Ezzie doesn't talk very much." Yes, I was a quiet child. I didn't talk very much. The reason at that time was my very strange belief that each person has a given number of words he could say in his lifetime. Apparently I was saving my allotment up for later. But later never came. I still am not an easy conversationalist. Yes, when I'm engaged in a discussion of my work or some subject I care deeply about, I will speak up. But I do not easily engage in "small talk."

If you wondered about the "Ezzie" reference above, my parents always called me "Ezzie," their English adaptation of a shortened version of Isadore.

What happened in 1919?

The 18th amendment to the U.S. Constitution was adopted, establishing prohibition; when Congress passed the Volstead Act to implement it, Wilson's veto was overridden.

The League of Nations was founded.
Benito Mussolini formed a fascist political movement in Italy.
Eugene V. Debs, a Communist, entered prison for opposing
the draft in wartime.
UCLA was founded.
The treaty of Versailles was signed; the U.S. Senate voted not to ratify it.
Afghanistan gained independence from the United Kingdom.
President Wilson suffered a stroke and was incapacitated.
The coal strike of 1919 occurred.

One strange event occurred on Biddle Street. Jewish kids can have a difficult time at Christmas. Although Chanukah did bring presents for the kids, observing Christmas presents for gentiles produced envy. Although my mother was very religious, one year she allowed us to hang stockings around Christmas/Chanukah time, and we received small token presents.

Years later I saw a newspaper article and photo describing President Carter's visit to a house that had been updated as part of a government rehab program. The address was 2251 E. Biddle Street—our former house.

I attended Clifton Park Junior High School. It was quite a distance from our house, but I walked each day, carrying heavy books back and forth under my arm (including a very large geography book). There were no backpacks then, or the wheeled book carts little kids trail behind them today.

We moved often, and we kids were never clued in about why or where we were going. I do recall that my mother often had disagreements with my father about the moves. That

> *Warren G. Harding served as president from 1921 to 1923.*

was the case in our second move. My belief is that we owned the house on Fleet Street where we lived first, and my father thought we could save on rent if we moved back there from Biddle Street. So we did move back for a short time. I do not think the business there went well.

What happened in the 1920s?

The 19th amendment to the U.S. Constitution granting voting rights to women was adopted.

The Chinese communist party was formed.

A worldwide smallpox epidemic occurred.

The N.Y. Yankees bought Babe Ruth.

The first commercial radio station in the U.S. started in Detroit.

The American Civil Liberties Union was established.

Walt Disney got his first job as an artist, paying $40 a week.

The League of Women Voters was formed.

Mahatma Gandhi was imprisoned.

Egypt gained its independence from Britain.

Hitler was sent to jail for barging in on a beer hall.

Charles Lindbergh was the first to fly solo across the Atlantic.

The Sacco Vanzetti trial took place.

Our next move was to 1807 E. Pratt Street, where my father gave up shoe repair and opened a grocery store. It was small and inefficient. The residence was reached by walking through a tunnel-like path to the rear.

We then moved to another grocery store, this one at 971 N. Chester Street. It was right next to an elevated train track. I recall helping in the store. We kept books when customers bought groceries without having the money in hand, a kind of credit system. I recall getting canned goods from the high shelves with a rod that had a scissors-like hook at the end. One incident there is memorable: Several of the boys were playing catch in the street next to the house. A policeman came by and charged us with a misdemeanor. I do not recall the outcome, but the experience was traumatic at the time.

The grocery business did not support the family. It was now about 1929—the depression. We were without sufficient funds. My parents learned of a place called "The Jewish Colony," supported by the Jewish Federation. We were what would today be called 'homeless.' We moved to the Colony, a farm community in the country. I have few recollections of that move, though this was surely the first time I learned about cows and milking.

My father bought a liquor store on South Broadway. I remember helping out on the Christmas-New Year holiday, when we did a rushing business.

Somehow my father learned about a restaurant that was for sale at 104 Market Place, about a block from the Pratt Street waterfront. We decided to buy it (where the funds came from I do not know). There was a residence on the second floor. What made this attractive? This was the period of Prohibition, the Federal law prohibiting the manufacture, possession, or sale of alcoholic beverages. What made this restaurant attractive was that it sold whiskey—mostly by the shot poured into a coffee mug, though we also sold half pints. The process was well rehearsed. There was the delivery to the store of a clear liquid in a five gallon glass jug. It was carried upstairs, where it was colored like whiskey by adding a caramel-like liquid. It was poured into half pint bottles for sale, or in a container from which shots could be poured behind a wood frame in the restaurant. The half-pint bottles were stored in the attic under floor boards that were loosened. We served full-course meals; my recollection is that we charged about $6 for such a meal.

Calvin Coolidge served as president of the U.S. from 1923 to 1929.

I was about 12 years old. I helped out in the restaurant, and I also helped in the kitchen. The chef was a "Negro" named Mr. Stewart. He taught me how to flip a fried egg or omelet, to fry a steak, and generally work as a second cook. We also advertised specials of the day on the front window of the restaurant. It was my job to write the specials on the glass with a white chalk-like liquid.

There was a man with a limp who hung around the restaurant whom we called Popcorn. My father worked out a deal with him to rent a horse and wagon and work as an "A-raber," hawking watermelons, fruits, and vegetables through the streets and alleys of the neighborhoods. I would occasionally ride with him.

The restaurant was right next door to an oyster shucking plant. We watched the skill with which the men shucked the oysters and packed them.

Many of the customers of the restaurant were sailors who came off months at sea with large rolls of bills after payday.

We did well financially for a time in the restaurant/liquor business. We did so well that my mother bought me a set of electric trains for Hanukkah. I was excited when we took them home and hooked them up. We turned on the power, and immediately saw smoke coming from the rheostat. We could not understand what happened. We took the set back to the store and asked what had happened. The storekeeper asked where we lived. When we told him we lived on Market Place, he said that explained the problem. The trains run on AC current; Market Place had DC current. He refused to make it good, and that ended my ownership of an electric train set. What disappointment.

Some time later Federal agents raided the restaurant and found the liquor. My father had a court appearance, and I believe that he paid a fine. We soon gave up the business. The man who sold us the business had signed an agreement that he would not open a similar restaurant within a set number of miles. A cousin of his opened such a restaurant a block from ours. We suspected that the former owner probably informed on us.

It was during the time we lived on Market Place that my father bought a *Baltimore Sun* paper route. We delivered the morning paper around 2 or 3 a.m. on an assigned route with designated customers. We placed the papers behind screen doors, on porches, on stoops, etc. I began assisting on this route about this time and continued it for several years. We also delivered the afternoon paper, and then collected on Saturdays. One part of the route where we delivered papers was the old Camden Station railroad—the site that is now the Orioles baseball stadium. One stop on my newspaper route was the home of an older black man who was blind. He bought several papers and resold them. I remember sitting listening to his tales of lifetime experiences. Another stop on our route was a funeral parlor. When I went in to collect and saw bodies in coffins, I can't quite describe accurately my feeling. It was fear, wonder, unpleasant. I got out as quickly as I could.

My father and my older brothers also delivered papers in the early morning. It was at this time, when I was about 13 or 14 years old, that I learned to drive our car—but only in the dead of nights and a few blocks.

One year the *Baltimore Sun* ran a contest for enrolling new subscribers to the paper. I entered and won a prize. Accompanied by my mother, I collected the prize—a pair of tan knickers that we obtained at a downtown department store.

It was during the period of my *Sunpaper* experience that I recall the *Sun* began to sponsor a radio program where it delivered the news. This was an experiment—would it help or damage circulation of the paper if people could hear the news on the radio?

I was apparently nurturing my interest in the theatre at this time, because on Saturdays when I was collecting on the newspaper route, I would collect a few dollars; buy a ticket at the Hippodrome, a movie house that also had a regular vaudeville show. I went every Saturday, then continued my collections for the newspaper when the show was over. The family knew nothing

about this. I was fascinated by the variety of performers--jugglers, comedians, dancers, specialty acts, magicians, acrobats. I recall one performance that demonstrated the predecessor of television; a camera on one side of the stage and a screen on the other side showing what was being seen by the camera.

We moved again, this time to Morrill Park at 1913 Cassadell Avenue. Pop rented a store in the business district of Morrill Park and continued his shoe repair and shoe store. We bought a large house not far away. It was the largest house we lived in to that time; it had three floors. This is

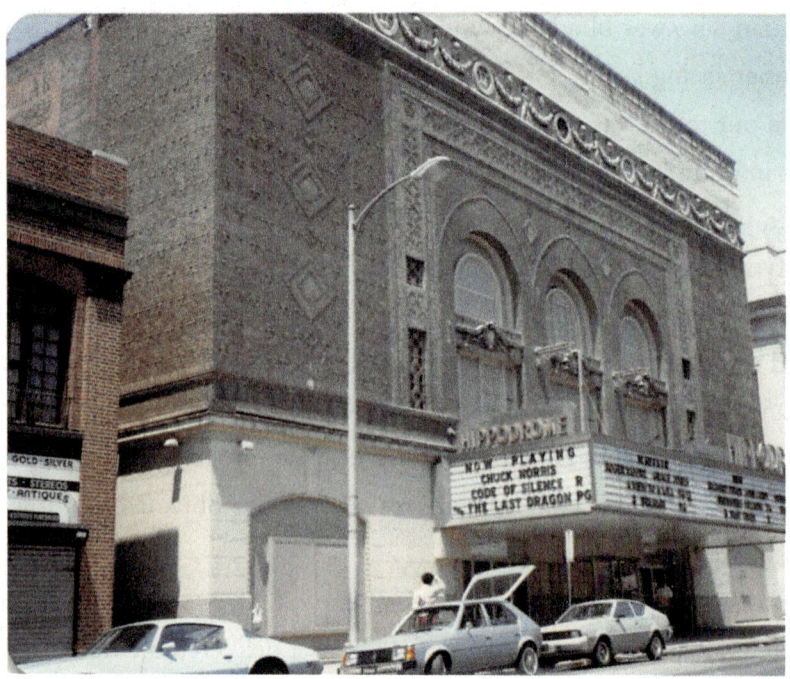

The Hippodrome Theatre.

where we had the twins as foster children.

I was now 13 years old; time for Bar Mitzvah. I have vague recollections of this affair. I believe it was held in the orthodox Bond Street shul. I recall studying the trope for chanting the "maftir" (the week's portion from the Torah). I can see myself standing on the bimah. I remember the "shamus" (the person designated to keep order) shushing children who misbehaved. After the service there was a very simple gathering with "schnapps" (whiskey) and perhaps some cake, a contrast with today's elaborate parties, with DJs, loud music and games. More than that I do not recall.

> *In 1929 Herbert Hoover was inaugurated as president of the United States and served until 1933.*

Again the shoe repair business did not support the family. We were desperate. One day my father disappeared without telling my mother where he was going. Days passed and we heard nothing; exactly how long it lasted I do not recall. Soon we learned that he had gone to Dayton, Ohio where he had a cousin who was in the shoe repair business. My father returned—I do not know how long after.

THE GREAT DEPRESSION

I was 13 years old when The Great Depression began in 1929. It started in the U.S. but soon became worldwide. It lasted until about the 1940s. Stock prices fell in September, but October 29, 1929 is known as Black Tuesday when the market crashed. International trade fell 50 percent. U.S. unemployment reached 25 percent; in some countries it was 33 percent. Cities were hard hit; crop prices fell 60 percent. More than 5,000 banks failed. A classic picture is that showing men selling apples on street corners; bread lines also were common.

There are many theories about the causes, and the debate continues. What role did free markets play, and what effect did government policies play? Herbert Hoover was U.S. President.

The turnaround began with the election of Franklin D. Roosevelt in 1932. He initiated bold measures, introducing the New Deal, a series of government initiatives—the National Recovery Act, the Civilian Conservation Corps, price codes, minimum wages, etc. Between 1933 and 1939 federal expenditures tripled. Recovery slowly occurred into the 1940s. The growth of manufacturing for World War II contributed to the recovery.

It was during this time that Jules began selling newspapers, standing on a corner on a busy part of Baltimore. He sold all three papers—the *Sun*, the *News*, and the *Post*, a pink tabloid. If my recollection is correct, the papers cost 2 cents each. I joined him some weekends. We not only sold on the corner, we also "hopped" on the streetcars (without paying a fare) and sold papers on the streetcar. Both of us were under the legal age for "working." A permit was required, and we were too young to get one. We were constantly afraid that the "badge man" would come by and ask to see our "badge" permit. I recall one cold winter day when Jules came home after a full Saturday on the corner, his feet almost frozen. My mother prepared a hot pan of water to soak his feet.

At about age 13, I got my first real job. My mother accompanied me to a confectionary and soda shop in the Morrill Park neighborhood, not far from our house. The owner agreed to hire me for after-school and weekend hours. I sold candy, prepared sodas, cleaned the store, and was otherwise general handyman. I recall the signs of my youth and immaturity. The owner asked me to sweep the floor. The next day he again asked me to sweep the floor. After repeating the instruction many times, he finally made it clear: I was supposed to sweep the floor each day when I arrived. My pay started at $2.50 a week; after a short time I got a raise.

We moved to a house at 2640 W. North Avenue. It was up on a hill, with two pairs of steps leading to the porch. I remember very little of this move.

Our tenth and final move was to the best house we ever lived in, at 2474 Shirley Avenue in the Park Heights section of Baltimore. It was a three-story bungalow, with a front porch that had a swing; there were flowers in the front, a lawn in the rear with fruit trees, and we owned several garage spaces in the rear alley. There was an upright piano that came with the house, and I learned to pick out tunes with one finger. Mef learned to play arias from operas as he and Will developed a life-long passion for opera. The public library was only a block away.

High School Years
1931-1933 (I was 15 to 17)

Public schools in Baltimore were segregated not only by race, but most high schools were also segregated by gender. I attended a high school called Baltimore City College, an all-male school. (Across the street was an all-female high school.)

I studied Latin, enjoyed math and English, but my real memory of high school is the beginning and enduring passion about drama and acting. Part of my English classes was drama, taught by Mr. Hecht. I tried out for a part in every play put on at school. I was in the junior play, and I was in every play put on in my senior year. I remember even playing a part in a play where I was only an offstage voice. At one point a student play was being broadcast on radio, and I got a part in that play—a fascinating experience for a young striving actor.

In the senior play, *The Queen's Husband* by Robert E. Sherwood, I played the part of the villain—General Northrup. I was intrigued by the uniform I wore, sword and all. The coach was Mr. Desch. I remember being a shy and less mature person than most of the others in the cast. The leading part in the play was played by Garrison Morfit. He later changed his name to Gary Moore, was spotted by Jimmy Durante and became part of his team, and later was the host of "I've Got a Secret" on TV. The queen was

> *In 1933 Franklin D. Roosevelt was inaugurated as president of the United States. He served until his death in 1944.*

played by William Rogers, one of the few names I remember from high school. The play was reviewed by the drama critic of the *Baltimore Sun* and I got a favorable mention in the article.

What happened in the 1930s?

Hitler became Chancellor of Germany. His troops marched into Austria and later Poland.
Mussolini invaded Ethiopia.
Japan invaded China.
King Edward VIII gave up the British throne to marry Wallace Simpson.
Franklin D. Roosevelt started his "fireside chats."
The Tennessee Valley Authority was formed.
The first commercial flight crossed the Atlantic.

Throughout my high school years I had no clear idea as to what profession I was interested in, other than acting. In my last year, thinking that I might become an industrial arts teacher, I took classes in wood-working and in printing. I remember setting type for the program for the senior play. It was interesting to set type for my own name in the program. I began to keep a scrap book of my acting experiences.

There were two other high school friends—Leonard Woolf and Herb Klein—with whom I continued an association after high school. During and after the high school years, when I lived on Shirley Avenue in the Park Heights area, I became a member of the Bialek Club. This club met at a Hebrew School not far from where I lived, and Leonard and Herb were also members. Our advisor was a teacher at the Hebrew School, Louis Schwartzman. He was a very friendly, stimulating, and challenging leader of the group. We studied Jewish history, engaged in debates with each other and other clubs, met sometimes with a girls club also meeting in the building, attended dances, and other social affairs.

The club disbanded after several years. About 30 or 40 years later, one of the members decided to bring the group together again. We met at a restaurant in Baltimore, and rehashed old times, told jokes, ate, and reported on major events in our lives. We continued to meet once a month, sometimes at Johns Hopkins Student Union. Finally, as members died or lost interest, the group disbanded again.

Two Years as a Vagabond (Player)
1933-1935 (I was 17 to 19)

I graduated from high school in 1933 at age 17. Except for my passion for acting and the theatre, I had no idea what I wanted to do. Ordinary college with a live-in dorm was never a serious consideration; it cost money we didn't have and none of my brothers had gone to a regular college.

As we were preparing to graduate from high school, my friend

William Rogers who played the leading female role in the senior play, informed me of an amateur community theatre downtown, called the Vagabond Players. Adults played the parts, but they had recently formed the Junior Vagabonds for younger actors. He and I ventured forth to try our luck. I was captivated by the place. It was a genuine theatre, with a well-equipped stage. (It clearly had previously been a stable for carriages and horses in earlier years.) The only paid staff was the technical director, Bill McLaughlin. He was assisted by Bob Dobson.

I tried out for a part in the play, *Scandalabra*, written by Zelda Fitzgerald, wife of F. Scott Fitzgerald, and I was cast as a lawyer. I began to attend rehearsals frequently and became acquainted with the technical staff. They could always use help, and I was ready to be of service. I helped to construct sets, paint them, and learned to use the switchboard and set the lights. I was spending almost every day at the theatre.

I continued serving the *Baltimore Sun* and collecting, thus bringing a minimal financial contribution to the family coffers. When a play was running in which I had no part, I would attend performances and help change the sets between acts. Soon I was assigned to run the switchboard. Thus I was spending days and nights at the theatre. I recall one night when the show ran late and there was work to be done after the performance. I think I got home about 2 a.m. and my mother was frantic.

I played the part of a butler in *The Importance of Being Earnest* by Oscar Wilde. After a time I was well known at the theatre, and I tried out for a role in a senior Vagabond production. I was cast as Jordan Morris in the play called *Granite*. It was a role of a middle-aged and gruff husband, with dramatic scenes. The play was reviewed by the drama critic of the *Baltimore Sun*, who wrote: "In the role of Jordan Morris, Isadore Seeman contributes a carefully pitched and admirably sustained performance."

In a play about a marathon dance, I played the part of Sam the barber. The stage crew had never grasped my name as Isadore; seeing that performance they began calling me Sam, a name that stuck with me in later years.

I played other roles. I kept a scrapbook, and the index of the first book lists 39 entries. I served as stage manager and as lighting director, always helping the stage crew. I continued my days and nights at the Vagabonds. Another group I played with was the Vanguard Players. The only time I ever earned any money was my participation with Bill McLaughlin in working on the scenery for a play produced by the Junior League. Questions were, of course, raised by my parents—how long could I spend this way, contributing so little to the family funds, and not furthering my education. When confrontations occurred, my brother Will came to my defense, and insisted that I be given this opportunity that I loved. Two years passed and I was still a Vagabond.

I was 17 years old, a very young member of the senior Vagabond Players; there were frequent comments about my young age when we were preparing for a performance in the make-up room. I cite one memorable experience during the Vagabond years. At the theatre I met a somewhat older man, L. Meyer Site, who spent time at the theatre. He lived independently and had a nice apartment just a few blocks from the theatre. I would often go with him to his apartment, listen to music, or just talk. I remember the feeling of independence that he displayed, and thought how nice it would be to have an apartment of my own.

Two years passed. I was in plays at the Young Men's and Young Women's Hebrew Association, and was head of their dramatic group for several years. What next? I was 19 years old. I recall sitting with my mother on the porch one day looking at the catalogue of the Baltimore College, a school with not a very high academic reputation, but a school frequented by working students. We reviewed a variety of possible courses, and my mother seemed to focus on the possibility of a course in advertising. We never followed this up.

Towson Teachers College
1936-1938 (I was 20 to 22)

O.K., I had a high school diploma and a taste of the amateur theatre world. What next? Will and Jules and even my younger brother Mef all advanced their education by attending Maryland State Teachers College at Towson, MD. It was the inexpensive way to an education and a career; living at home, thus no dorm costs, and very low tuition. They traveled to school on street cars, or by hitching rides. Even though I had felt no special interest in teaching school, it seemed the natural thing for me to follow the family pattern and register at Towson Teachers College. In 1935 I enrolled there for a three-year program, leading to a teaching certificate.

The principal at Teachers College was Lida Lee Toll, an elderly woman with restrictive instincts and practices. The atmosphere at the school was dull and traditional. I found most of the courses and teachers to be dull and not very challenging. There were two exceptions: the course and the instructor of the science class were exciting, and the teacher of the geography class was stimulating and amusing. I did not work very hard there, and my grades generally reflected that practice. All students were required to spend two semesters in "practice teaching" also called "student teaching" in the Baltimore public schools. I found this to be challenging and interesting, and I was graded A in these adventures. (Coincidentally, one of the practice teaching assignments was at School No. 6 which was just two blocks from where Shirley, later my wife, lived, and the school she attended, though at that time I did not know her.)

One of the rewarding experiences at Teachers College was the camaraderie in what was called "The Men's Room." It was not the lavatory, but rather a "social hall" for the men at the College. We would spend time there between classes and get acquainted with other male students.

I developed several close friendships there: with Leonard Woolf, Herb Klein, Siggie Spritz (who, because of the Seeman in my name always called me "Matey"), Bernard Gammerman, and others. There were frequent discussions there, and I recall one student named Charles Leaf who was a Communist who espoused the Soviet Union position on all matters political.

I remember one incident that called for a judgment on personal honesty, for me and for other students. The class was given a test, and the next day another class in the same subject was given the same test. The second day the teacher asked if any of us had conferred with students in the previous day's class about the questions on the test. In fact, several of us had, including me. We confessed to it. I do not recall the penalty, but several of us honestly confessed.

DIRECTOR OF DRAMATICS FOR THE BALTIMORE BOARD OF JEWISH EDUCATION 1934-1939 (I WAS 18 TO 23)

While at Teachers College I continued serving the *Baltimore Sun,* and continued my participation in plays around the Baltimore region. There was no program in dramatics at the college that I could participate in. I played Banquo in Shakespeare's *Macbeth* and played in *The Front Page.* Among the dramatic parts I played were some plays about the Jewish Holidays.

One year I played the part of Mattathias, the patriarch in the Chanukah story. It was held at the Lyric Theatre, the large theatre used for opera, symphonies, and other serious events. I received very favorable comments on the performance.

A short time later, I received a letter from Dr. Louis L. Kaplan, president of the Baltimore Board of Jewish Education, and a very well-known and respected leader of the Baltimore Jewish community. He wrote: "I want to thank you most warmly for all of your help in making

Sunday's entertainment so enjoyable. Without your voice and your excellent pointers with regards to staging and lighting, much of the dignity and color of the pantomimes would have been lost. When you are next in the neighborhood, I would appreciate your dropping in to see me as I would like to talk to you about several matters." I arranged an appointment and he invited me to become Director of Dramatics for the Board, a new position, with responsibility for directing plays about the Jewish holidays at the various Hebrew Schools affiliated with the Board of Jewish Education. I was excited to accept. The assignment was one I could carry out while attending school, since it involved meeting with the children and rehearsing after school. I found some plays that I could direct, and when I could not find a play I liked, I began to write my own plays for the holidays. I conferred with the principals of each school I worked at. I recruited children and they tried out for their roles. I coached them, managed simple scenery, and produced plays at a number of Hebrew Schools. One of the schools where I put on a play was the Har Zion Hebrew School on North Avenue, and one of the performers was a girl named Ada Rhea Cohen. (More of that later).

I took part in other plays at the time I was attending Teachers College. It was at that time that I became acquainted with a fellow actor with whom I became quite friendly. His name was David Kurland, more than a few years my senior, and a very accomplished actor. We were in several plays together, and I saw him perform in a Chekov play, *Uncle Vanya,* at Hopkins where he did an outstanding performance. Uncle Vanya cries at the close of the play. And Dave had real tears.

Summers at Hilltop Lodge
1938-1939 (I was 22 to 23)

Dave Kurland was chosen as one of the company of actors to perform on the social staff during the summer at a resort in the Catskills called "Hilltop Lodge." It was on Sylvan Lake. There was a main house, small cabins, and a social hall. Dave arranged for me to be invited to join the group as an assistant on the backstage crew, handling scenery, lighting, stage manager, properties, etc. I was pleased to accept.

Dave and I shared a cabin. I enjoyed the summer, though I had some problem with my boss, the scene designer. I felt that he did not give me enough rein to do things on my own; he assigned tiny specific jobs, rather than making a general assignment that I could carry out. There was enough other pleasure in the summer experience to overcome that issue.

It was at Hilltop Lodge that I had my first kiss. The resort was well known as a place that women from New York who were not yet married came to look for a mate, and men came to find a woman. I was too young and inexperienced for that, but I did find my first infatuation. I met a young woman from New York, Edith Joan Rothenberg, and we had dates together. We sat on adjacent swings, we went rowing on the lake, we walked around the lake, and we kissed; no more. When the summer was over, I corresponded with her. I went to a stationer and had letterhead prepared with a design of her initials. I visited her once in New York. The next summer I met another young woman, Geraldine, and had a similar relationship. I visited her once in New York. At that time I began writing poetry, a practice I continued throughout my life.

Sam Sat In Sunnyside

Spring saw Sam Seeman in Sunnyside.
Sam saw GT.
Slowly they strolled to 47th Street,

Stood on the stair, and stared.
Soon they sat—and the sofa sank.
So they stood, to serve and to sup.
To step outside to see the sun and the stars,
The shows the city was selling.
They sat again as the subway sped
Then swiftly to Sunnyside.
Soon they sat and the sofa sank.
Softly they spoke, sat silently still.
But they stayed on the sofa, still slowly sinking,
Sat as the sofa sank.

I've a song to sing, and a story to say
Of a sinking sofa in Sunnyside.
Of speaking and sighing and soft caress,
A song of sincere affection.
Of sharing and living, a song of life—
So sweetly, sing with me this song of Sam
And the sinking sofa in Sunnyside.

Dave Kurland had different ambitions. One night he asked me to stay out of the cabin until one a.m. I knew why.

The second year I was there I was able to arrange for my brother Will to come with me and serve as a waiter

These years in the theatre—these experiences—are clearly the most memorable and most exhilarating times of my early life. I was accepted as a competent actor, and a decent human being. The process of being invited and trying out successfully at a variety of theatre groups, and serving the Board of Jewish Education, was rewarding. I developed a system for learning my lines and shaping the character of the part I was playing. The applause of the audience was very gratifying. My days rehearsing and evenings performing were most satisfying. I remember feeling that an evening spent at home made an incomplete day.

A Two-Year Teacher
1938-1940 (I was 22 to 24)

I graduated from Towson Teachers College in June 1938 at age 22 with a three-year diploma and a teaching certificate. It was the practice at that time for teaching graduates to apply for a job in the Baltimore Public Schools, and to take an exam that graded you, placing you on a list of priorities for openings in the system. (I recall that Will scored first on the list, but it was during the depression and the economy was so bad that all he could get was daily jobs as a substitute when regular teachers were ill or otherwise absent.)

I scored high enough to be placed, and began teaching the sixth grade at the elementary school on the campus of Baltimore City College where I had attended high school. It was not a very nice neighborhood, and I soon discovered that there was more effort to maintain discipline in the class than there was actual teaching. I taught all subjects: arithmetic, reading, geography, history, penmanship, and even music and art, though ill prepared for these latter subjects.

It was at that time that all four Seeman brothers were teachers in the Baltimore City Public Schools. I recall the four of us sitting in the second balcony at the Ford's Theatre in Baltimore, a regular sight for the four Seeman boys to be seen about the city.

I cite one example to show how discipline overpowered teaching. I had one female student who was physically well developed as a sixth grader and a very troublesome presence in the classroom. There was a cloakroom at the rear of the class. One day this girl went in to the cloakroom and used her cigarette lighter to set fire to the fur collar on another student's coat. I reported this and other incidents to my supervisor with a recommendation that she be evaluated as a mental health problem. She was evaluated, and they simply returned her to my classroom.

Meeting Shirley
1939 (I was 23)

While spending the days teaching, I followed the practice of my brothers in taking night-school classes to advance our education, since we did not yet have a degree. I enrolled at Johns Hopkins University night school and took courses in Shakespeare, drama, archaeology, and world history.

One evening I received a telephone call from a girl who was also taking the world history course at Hopkins. The class had been assigned a textbook, but copies were not readily available. I had a copy, she did not. She called to ask if we could study together. I readily agreed. We arranged to meet after class the next day. We did not attempt to describe each other, and she later wondered how I identified her. I am not sure how I did, but I did, and we rode home together on the street car part of the way. Her name was Shirley Cohen. She later explained to me how she knew me. She identified me as the dramatics coach at the Hebrew School where her younger sister Ada Rhea had been in one of my plays. That

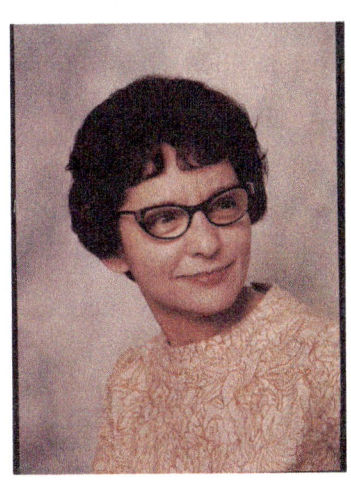

Shirley

was the beginning of more than 63 years together.

We began to study together, often at her house. There I met her sister—Ada Rhea Cohen, of my drama coaching days. I met her parents, her brother Irvin, and her sister Evelyn. Shirley and I studied together, and rode the street car together, but we also became romantically involved. I sometimes had the use of the family car, and we would drive into the country. Or we would sit in her living room, study, and later just "neck." When my brothers were getting ready to go out on dates, it was always clear who I was going out with. We attended theatre and concerts together. We were "girlfriend" and "boyfriend." We often met at the main public library downtown and listened to music in the special music room. She met my family. It was clear that we were serious.

TUBERCULOSIS CHANGES MY LIFE

In the summer of 1941 two of my brothers and I drove over to Washington to attend a session at the U.S. Senate. While sitting in the Senate gallery, I began to spit up some blood (a condition I later learned to call hemoptysis). My brothers took me to the office of the capitol physician, who examined me and advised me to go home immediately and to see my physician. I did so and was referred to a lung specialist, who took chest x-rays. He informed me that there was a small spot on the lungs that needed to be watched.

That summer I had arranged to serve as a stage hand at a summer resort in Pennsylvania. I went there, and after a week or so, I spit up blood again. I came home soon thereafter and again saw the lung specialist. He concluded that I had tuberculosis, and arranged for me to be admitted to Mt. Pleasant, a tuberculosis sanatorium operated by the Associated Jewish Charities of Baltimore. It was located in Reisterstown, a few miles outside of Baltimore.

The sanatorium experience proved to be life-changing for me. I was placed in a bed on a ward on an outside porch with perhaps ten other patients. My treatment was to be complete bed rest. At that time there were no drugs known to treat tuberculosis. The only treatments were bed rest, or pneumothorax (called pneumo by patients), in which air is introduced into the lung to collapse it so that it can heal itself, or thoracoplasty, in which some ribs were cut to enable the lungs to collapse and heal. There were regular sputum tests to determine if the tubercle bacillus was present. There were also periodic chest x-rays. Meals were served in bed. My condition did permit me to go to the bathroom. Otherwise, it was twenty-four hours a day lying in bed outside on the porch, summer and winter, rain or shine.

The "social" system on the porch was quite interesting. Since virtually all of the patients were on bed rest, there was not much direct personal exchange. We had one regular nurse, Miss Wylie. She was attentive, but with not a great bedside manner. She was somewhat of a prude. There was one patient who was on pneumothorax and thus able to walk around. He was called Abe; a short, stout, verbose man, who constantly teased Miss Wylie, and she responded in kind. He spent much time in the pottery room making small vases from molds. Before I left Mt. Pleasant I made a vase from one of his molds.

Shirley did not have a car. My brother Will agreed to teach her how to drive, and when she obtained her license, my parents agreed to let her use our car to visit me. I was able to get up and sit with her in the library. I wrote to her every day, and she wrote often.

My brothers would visit me at the sanitarium, and since my mother did not drive, Will often brought her there. Will visited often, and he began to undertake the serious education of his younger brother. He brought me books regularly—books on logic, on philosophy, on politics, on history—serious books for study, not for pleasure reading. I swallowed them eagerly. I read them and took notes on them. I was growing in my perspective of the world.

With time as my greatest asset, and lying in bed outdoors following the track of the sun and the moon and the stars and the clouds, there was much opportunity to think and reflect.

I began writing poetry, serious and light.

The Ballad of TB

Sing for T, and sing for B,
Sing tubercle bacillus.
We're on the cure and mighty sure
We'll live, though it may kill us.

I recall hoping at each sputum test and x-ray exam that I would be found free of the disease and ready for discharge. I believed all along that it was a mild case of TB. I began reading *The Magic Mountain*, a book about tuberculosis, but it was very dull, and I gave up. I did read all I could about TB and wrote poems about TB.

Song of the Cure

If things look dark and you desperately decide
It's time for the end, and you choose suicide,
The knife's in your hand; too late, with one stride –
    Look out, you fool, it's your pneumo side.
If the doctors say you're negative
Because you really tried
To brave the zero weather
While the rest stayed inside,
And your chest begins to swell in justifiable pride--
    Look out, you fool, it's your pneumo side.

When you're finally discharged, and you step outside,
And you feel you're free, once again your own guide,
With one fell gesture you fling your arms wide--
    Look out, you fool, it's your pneumo side.

When you meet the girl you love,
And you're close beside

The dear one you've asked to be your bride,
She sighed, and replied, and your arms begin to glide—
Look out, you fool, it's your pneumo side.

I don't know at what point it occurred, but since I had not until then known what I wanted as my career (other than a vain hope of being a professional actor), I began to think of a career in public health. How does one chose his or her life's work? It requires some passion. No one, I felt, needs to get tuberculosis; public health can prevent communicable diseases. That was what I chose.

With so much time spent just lying in bed, my thoughts turned to reflections on life, on philosophy, on existence.

Credo

Within the compass of time's hourly round,
Ere each his neighbor hour urges on,
My student soul, from eyes that look upon
Both men whose deepest vision hugs the ground
And those whose noble zeal can know no bound,
From ears attuned to melody and moan,
Does learn the spotless angels' wings to don,
And hasten then the depths of hell to sound.

You men who would be deemed worth your life,
Ere you have spent your mortal span on earth,
Set down your purpose--serve as you'd be served.
Relentless, then, achievement take to wife,
Succeeding, you have paid your price of birth.
Then is joy just and happiness deserved.

Time moved slowly, lying in bed day and night.

No Monument Marks the Day

No monument marks the day.

> *Unheeding time winds off her endless spool,*
> *Casting to men below*
> > *The formless, shapeless stuff that is herself*
> > *To reckon up and file away in clock and calendar.*

This is the day, as men do reckon it,
> *Since last I knew the world as home.*
> *This spot of earth that is my bed*
> > *Hath half of heaven circled,*
> > *And charted out the course of sun and stars.*

Full half a year hath turned.
> *Day neighbor night's successor, then lives out her own*
> *Well counted hours, and is sent*
> > *Below the earth, into eternal nothingness,*
> > *New night succeeding newer days.*

And thus has this day come.
> *No monument marks the day.*
> *Simply, I pause, and look into the chart*
> > *Of days gone by, and days to come,*
> > *And search for the meaning of time.*

Fourteen months after I was admitted to Mt. Pleasant I was discharged.

TB Limerick

There was a tubercular gent
Who died of astonishment.

The bugs that had clung
To the hole in his lung,
Were gone. He had coughed 'till they went.

World War II

In 1939 Germany, under Adolph Hitler's rule, invaded Poland,
and World War II began. The Allies opposed the Axis, and the war
continued until 1945. More than 100 million military personnel were
mobilized. There were between 50 million and 70 million fatalities. In
the Battle of Britain, German planes attacked the United Kingdom.
The Holocaust was perpetrated by Germany. On December 7, 1941 the
Japanese attacked the U.S. at Pearl Harbor, and the U.S. entered the
war.

Germany surrendered on May 8, 1945. After atomic bombs were
dropped on two Japanese cities, Japan surrendered on August 15, 1945.
The United Nations was established to avert future wars.

WORLD WAR II AND THE DRAFT
1941 (I WAS 25)

The United States entered World War II near the close of 1941 after
the Japanese attack on Pearl Harbor. The Selective Training and Service
Act was passed in 1940 by Congress, drafting all eligible men ages 18 to
45. We were required to register with our local Draft Board. I registered
while I was at Mt. Pleasant and was classified IV-F, ineligible because of
health.

The Act provided for men who could satisfactorily prove that they
were conscientious objectors (CO) to serve in Civilian Public Service instead of military service. My brother Will was the first of us to be called,
and he filed for conscientious objector status. He had carefully prepared
his case, knowing that it would be difficult for a Jew to be accepted into

this category. Quakers and other religious groups that were known to oppose war were rather easily granted CO status. Jews were not. Will was initially turned down, but on appeal he prevailed. He was first sent to a Civilian Public Service Camp in West Compton, New Hampshire. He volunteered to take part in an experiment in which lice were sown into the underpants of participants and DDT powder was used to eradicate them. At another time on Welfare Island in New York he enrolled in an experiment testing the effect of diets on the ability to be sustained in high altitudes. When he realized this experiment served a military purpose, he dropped out of the experiment. Later, before he completed his service, he worked in a bakery at a hospital in New York.

Mef also filed as a conscientious objector and he also was initially denied CO status. He appealed and after an investigation by the FBI, he was granted IV-E status as a CO. He was assigned to a Civilian Public Service Camp in Coshocton, Ohio, an abandoned Civilian Conservation Corps Camp from the Roosevelt days. The task was to assist nearby farmers in preparing hilly land for use as strip-farming. Later he was assigned administrative duty because of problems with physical activity. Jules also filed as a CO, but as the time approached to begin service he became emotionally ill and spent some time in a hospital. He was granted IV-F status because of illness.

When I was discharged from Mt. Pleasant I reported to my Draft Board. Oddly enough they reclassified me as I-A, eligible to serve. I appealed and they recognized the absurdity of this action and reclassified me a IV-F for health reasons. In the meantime I, too, had filed papers as a conscientious objector, but was never required to defend this position.

What happened in the 1940s?

Japan attacked Pearl Harbor.
Leon Trotsky was assassinated.
Anne Frank went into hiding and wrote her diary.
Japanese Americans were sent to internment camps.

FDR died.
D-Day, the invasion of Europe, occurred.
Hitler committed suicide.
Atomic bombs were dropped on Hiroshima and Nagasaki.
The United Nations was formed.

After discharge from the sanatorium, I returned to work in teaching. I had now made up my mind that I wanted a career in public health and not in teaching elementary school. I worked for two months and resigned.

A NEW CAREER
1942 (I WAS 26)

In the meantime I began seeking ways to enter public health. I wrote to the National Tuberculosis Association and to other national health organizations, but received no encouragement. I decided on a long shot and went to the office of the Baltimore City Health Department. Fortune was on my side.

I went to the office of the Commissioner of Health, but fortunately he was not in at the time. I told his secretary what I was seeking and she referred me to the Deputy Commissioner of Health, Dr. Ross Davies.

He listened to my appeal for a job in the department and took serious interest in helping me. Since it was clear that I had no experience, he tried to identify the kinds of jobs in the department that I might qualify for without a degree. He suggested some work in the laboratory, or becoming trained as a sanitary inspector. He then remembered that the person who occupied the position of Chief Clerk in the office of the Bureau of Vital Statistics was retiring and suggested that I speak with the director of the bureau. He called him and advised him that I would meet with him about the position.

I met with Dr. W. Thurber Fales who described the work. He planned to establish a position as administrative assistant in the bureau; it entailed supervising the clerical staff and helping in managing the work of the bureau.

He agreed to submit my name in application for the position to the Civil Service office. It worked; I got the job. It paid the great sum of $2,400 a year.

MARRIAGE
1942 (I WAS 26)

Shirley and I had kept up our close relationship through the Mt. Pleasant months and after. We were never formally engaged but it became clear that we intended to marry.

Is there a common process where one or both members of a couple make a decision that marriage is the choice? Having married only once, I cannot speak personally about whatever the general process of deciding that one will marry occurs. I know that during the afternoons and evenings that Shirley and I sat next to each other on the sofa in her living room and studied, and held each other, and kissed, I had thoughts about where this was heading. Shirley had a beautiful smile. She had a keen intellect. She had a wide curiosity. She was ever eager for education. And she obviously felt close to me.

At the same time, I was well aware of the continuing troubling effect of her early years of living with a tyrannical, ultra-religious father incapable of showing love for his children, and a caring mother but one who made her daughter feel unaccepted and inadequate. At some point I decided that I could show her that my love for her would lead to a happy lifelong relationship for both of us.

One time during this period we struck out on an adventure both strange and daring for an unsophisticated and shy unmarried couple. We took a trip to New York City to see an opera at the Metropolitan Opera. I bought tickets in the highest balcony. We reserved separate rooms in a very modest hotel, and while I did visit her in her room at night, I did not sleep with her or spend the night in her room. I kept on the lookout for the hotel detective. Since this was to be a great adventure for us, we had dinner before the opera in an expensive restaurant—Longchamps. When I looked at the menu prices, my heart sank. I could see myself washing the dishes after the meal. With careful selection of our meals at the lowest prices, I was barely able to pay the check.

Shirley had worked as a secretary on several jobs: for the Jewish Family and Children's Bureau, for a clothing manufacturer, at the Census Bureau, and at Edgewood Arsenal as secretary to a military officer. Now that I had a responsible position, we could seriously take the step. We were married on October 18, 1942. An interesting side note: Shirley's cousin Sylvan Wolpert planned to be married on October 25, and we had originally planned our wedding on the same date. Sylvan wanted to avoid a conflict for some relatives, and asked us to change our date, so we accommodated and chose October 18. In later years, I sometimes had difficulty remembering our wedding day--October 25 or 18?

We were married in the living room of Rabbi Nathan Drazen on Auchentorily Terrace in Baltimore. It was as modest a ceremony as one can conceive, with only our immediate families present. I recall my father was unimpressed and came wearing a pair of sloppy pants. We rented a third-floor apartment in the home of a distant relative of Shirley's.

One evening before the wedding we were talking with Shirley's parents about the wedding. They ardently

Left: Shirley as a child. Right: Shirley and her mother.

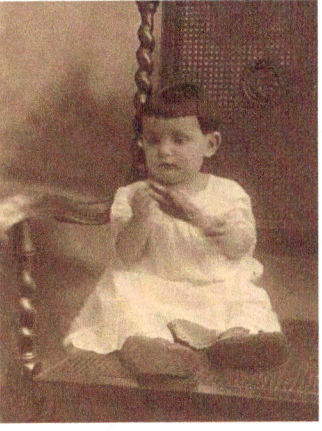
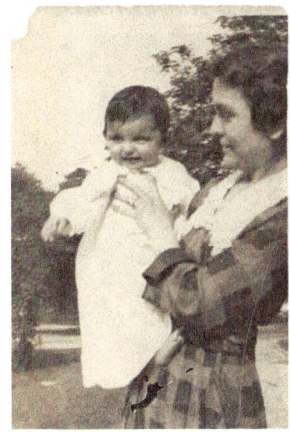

pleaded with us to keep a kosher home, but we made it clear we had no intention to do so. Shirley's father was an exceedingly religious man, observing Jewish laws very strictly, and imposing them on his children. Shirley had an older brother, Irvin, who had attended Jewish day school. As he became adolescent he broke away from the religious mode, and since he was close to Shirley, she followed suit. Shirley never recovered from the early oppressive and fanatical religious experience and for the remainder of her life had difficulty finding a satisfactory accord with religion.

We did not have the resources, the time, or the inclination to go on a honeymoon. Instead, some months after our marriage we took a bus to a small city near Frederick, Maryland. We rented a room in a very modest vacation accommodation for a week. When we got there, we realized our poor selection. Most of the vacationers were much older, sitting on the porch rocking much of the day. We did some walking and were able to take trips into Frederick, but hardly a very exciting getaway.

AT THE BALTIMORE CITY HEALTH DEPARTMENT

The new job proved to be very engrossing, challenging, and a great introduction to the public health field. Dr. Fales was a wonderful role model, supervisor, and friend. With the guidance and support he pro-

Shirley's grandparents.

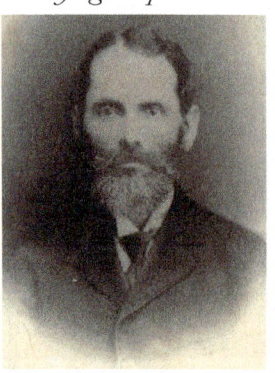
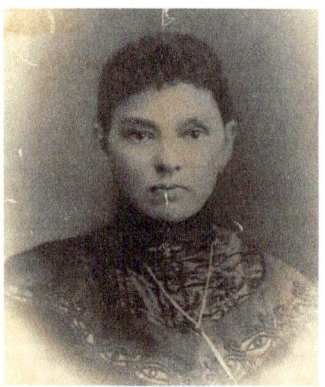

vided to me, I often characterize him as a second father. He was very competent, professional, involved in community affairs, and friendly. He worked closely with Dr.

Lowell Reed, an outstanding leader in public health statistics, and professor at the Johns Hopkins School of Hygiene and Public Health. I took a course in statistics with Dr. Reed.

The Bureau of Vital Statistics had two primary functions: it served as the registration office for births and deaths in Baltimore City, and it was the statistical center for public health events in the city. My primary duties initially centered on the vital records function. There was a staff of about 15 clerks whom I supervised. We registered all births and deaths in the city, with many contacts with funeral directors who registered the deaths.

The country was participating in World War II, with a great emphasis on production of weapons for war. In order to gain employment in the war effort, one had to prove citizenship. The best way to do that was to produce a birth certificate, so we were selling certified copies of birth records like hotcakes. In addition to hunting for the records, we were involved in correction of existing records, and completing Delayed Certificates of Birth for persons for whom no birth records was found, but could provide clear evidence of birth in the city, e.g., school records, insurance records, baptismal records, etc. Another large part of the work involved selling copies of death certificates for insurance purposes and estate matters.

I was also interested in the statistical function of the office. I devoted some effort to examining the birth data and wrote several articles which were published in magazines such as baby magazines. In my effort in the statistical function of the office which Dr. Fales had developed extensively, working with other offices in the Health Department and with many community groups, while I worked with the several clerks assigned to statistics. We prepared an 80-column IBM punch card for each birth and death recorded, and we had a counting sorter, a Hollerith machine, to analyze the data. Dr. Fales had expressed an interest in the study of death certificates that listed multiple causes of death, and under his guidance, I prepared an article on multiple causes. I also became involved in meetings of the National Office of Vital Statistics in the U. S. Public Health Service. I recall accompanying Dr. Fales on a trip to Chicago for such a meeting, my first trip to Chicago, and meeting Dr. Halbert L. Dunn, the head of the Office.

> *In 1944 Harry S. Truman became president of the United States after the death of Roosevelt. Truman was inaugurated on April 1945 after his own election.*

It was on this trip to Chicago that I was introduced to a lifestyle new to me. It was the first time I stayed in an expensive hotel, my first attendance at a national professional conference, and most memorable, a steak so delicious, tasty, and tender that I have yearned for such a one ever since.

FURTHER EDUCATION FOR SHIRLEY AND ME
1943-1944 (I WAS 27 TO 28)

I did not yet have a Bachelor's degree, since Teachers College was only a three-year course, and my work at Hopkins had brought my total education credits up to 119. I was well aware that a fruitful career required a Bachelor's and an advanced degree. In consultation with Dr. Fales, I arranged to enroll at Teachers College at Columbia University to complete my Bachelor's degree. I also sought the opportunity to sit in on some classes at the School of Public Health at Columbia, but I was not accepted. I made a commitment to return to the department for at least two years.

Shirley had developed an interest in nursery school teaching in place of the secretarial work she had done previously. Before we were married, she had found a position as an aide in a nursery school in Silver Spring, Maryland. The school was located in a private house on Colesville Road. I visited her in Silver Spring on several occasions. Later she found a position at the Park School in Baltimore. She was interested in further training. She and I had discussions about my plan to go to Columbia University and she decided to enroll at the Bank Street College of Education in New York for training as a nursery school teacher.

Shirley went to New York ahead of me and found a one-room apartment on W. 104th Street, with a $35 monthly rental. There was a bedroom-living room, and a bathroom. In the hall there was a refrigerator and a hotplate for cooking. Shirley took the subway to Bank Street; I usually walked to Columbia. We ate out often, either at the automat or a cheap restaurant on upper Broadway. We attended a few plays, but money was scarce. We borrowed some money from Will and from my parents to finance the adventure. At that time the national headquarters of the American Public Health Association was located in New York. I applied there and was given a part-time job calculating data for a national publication, Local Health Units for the Nation. APHA was also developing tests to certify public health workers and invited members to submit questions for the tests, for which they paid a modest fee. I submitted quite a few questions which were accepted. While we were in New York, Will had two Civilian Public Service assignments there, in a hospital bakery and the diet study, so he visited us often. He was also in therapy at the time.

In spite of our lack of adequate financial resources, Shirley and I decided to purchase a professional portrait. It is one of my prize possessions.

While we were in New York we learned that Shirley's mother was very ill; she had a fistula in the rectum, and it was diagnosed as due to acute myeloid leukemia.

I completed work for my B.S. degree and Shirley completed her course at Bank Street. (I got an A in all of my courses.)

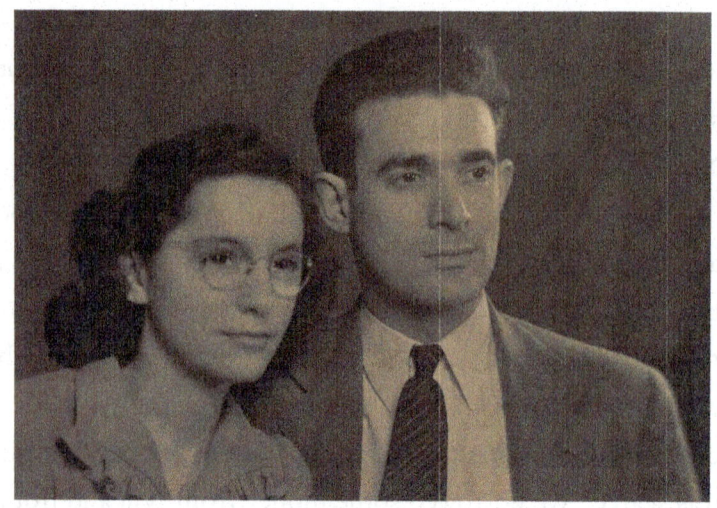

Shirley and me, taken in New York, pensive.

BACK TO BALTIMORE; SHIRLEY'S MOTHER DIES
1944

We returned to Baltimore and rented a second-floor apartment on Beehler Avenue. Very soon after we returned, Shirley's mother was hospitalized with a diagnosis of acute leukemia. We visited her, and we were in the hospital the day she died. This was a major blow to the Cohen family. Irvin was teaching in Boston and Ada Rhea was married. That left Shirley's father Ralph and her youngest sister Evie alone in the Smallwood Street house. That could not last very long. We found a family who kept kosher and had a room to rent, and her father, Ralph, moved in. Evie moved to New York where she got a job and where her friend Murray Weingarten lived.

With my interest in public health, Shirley's mother's death led me to examine statistics on mortality from leukemia. I consulted Dr. Milton Sacks, a physician at the University of Maryland, and together we wrote an article on trends in mortality from leukemia in the U.S. We were successful in having it published in *Blood, the Journal of Hematology*. This was my first professional journal article.

RETURN TO THE BALTIMORE CITY HEALTH DEPARTMENT
1944-1946

Now with a B.S.degree, I returned to the Health Department and Shirley found a nursery school position. Soon after, Dr. Fales was eager to reorganize the Bureau of Vital Statistics so that he could receive a higher pay. He created the Statistical Section, a higher level unit, and within it he created a Bureau of Vital Records and a Bureau of Vital Statistics. He arranged to appoint me as Director of the Bureau of Vital Records. He found no satisfactory candidate to head the other bureau, so I also maintained my interest in the statistical work of the office. I had some contacts with the Commissioner of Health, Dr. Huntington Williams. He was a strong leader with a firm grip on all of the work of the department. I recall one meeting in his office when he was vigorously announcing his insistence about the size of type to be required on the cap of milk bottles recording the fact that the milk was pasteurized and listing the expiration date.

NUCLEAR WEAPONS

In 1942 during World War II President Roosevelt authorized a program to develop a nuclear bomb, and this program continued under President Truman. It was known as the Manhattan Project, centered in Los Alamos, and headed by Robert Oppenheimer. It was known that Germany was also attempting to develop a nuclear weapon.

In July 1945 the first bomb was successfully tested. President Truman authorized the military to drop an atomic bomb on Hiroshima in Japan on August 6, 1945 and another on Nagasaki on August 9, 1945. Soon after, the Japanese surrendered, ending World War II.

The Soviet Union tested its first atomic bomb in August 1949, and the atomic arms race was begun. Over time more than 2,000 bomb tests were held. Both the U.S. and the Soviets developed inter-continental ballistic missiles to deliver atomic bombs to the enemy. Other nations developed the bomb, including the United Kingdom, France, China, India, Pakistan and North Korea. It is believed that Israel has bombs, but it has never been acknowledged. In 1962 the United States observed atomic weapons in Cuba, delivered by the Soviet Union. It was the Cuban Missile Crisis. President Kennedy demanded that they be removed, and after a tense period, the Soviets agreed.

There have been many efforts at control. In 1963 a Partial Test Ban Treaty was signed. In 1972 an Anti-Ballistic Missile Treaty was signed.

A GRADUATE DEGREE
1946-1947 (I WAS 30 TO 31)

I continued working for the Health Department for three years when I decided it was time to go for a higher degree. I knew that a successful career required more than a B.S., especially with three brothers with PhDs.

In consultation with Dr. Fales, I explored The Johns Hopkins School of Hygiene and Public Health, but they had no major in health education which was the field I wanted to pursue. We decided on the School of Public Health at the University of Michigan. With his help I arranged to receive a very modest scholarship from the U.S. Public Health Service, with a promise to return to the department for two years.

To qualify for admission I had to take a course in chemistry, which I had not taken in high school, so I took the course at Johns Hopkins night school. I also needed a course in biology so I enrolled at the School of Nursing at the University of Maryland, where we dissected a cat in the course on Comparative Vertebrate Morphology.

A sidelight on this educational episode: since I had limited time between work and the evening class, I had a quick dinner downtown. I always managed to eat close to a restaurant that served delicious chocolate cupcakes—a favorite desert of mine. I'm not sure I have ever found their match.

Shirley flew out to Ann Arbor before I did and arranged to stay at the Michigan Union for several days, looking for an apartment. I also stayed at the Union when I arrived. I recall that Shirley was required to go in and out by a side door, since women could not use the front door at the Union.

She found a second floor unit in a house that accommodated students at 522 North Division Street. We had one room and a small narrow alcove where we placed a hot-plate. We shared a common bathroom on this floor with other students, with no running water in our apartment. To refrigerate milk and eggs I hung an egg crate outside our window. Shirley also arranged a position as nursery school teacher in Ann Arbor. This helped finance our Michigan stay.

I enrolled in courses in health education, statistics, public health administration, epidemiology, and tuberculosis. In connection with the administration course we had an assignment to spend several weeks in a local health department. I was assigned to Allegan County and I prepared an analysis of the county which won high praise from the instructor. I recall attending a Kiwanis Club meeting in the county, and I won the door prize.

In connection with the course in tuberculosis, I was the only non-MD taking the course. We observed an autopsy (Ugh!) and we observed a patient under therapy. I took statistics courses both semesters. (I got all A's in my courses at Michigan.) I was elected to the Public Health Honor Society and bought a pin.

I walked to school each day, and Ann Arbor was really cold in winter. I wore a wool cap and scarf. We walked everywhere. We ate out often at a very inexpensive restaurant or at the student cafeteria. We were introduced to chamber music with performances by the Guarneri String Quartet. We became quite friendly with a young couple with young twin boys. .

The Ann Arbor experience was memorable for many reasons, among them Shirley's pregnancy. She had difficulty with staining but overcame the problem.

BACK TO BALTIMORE AND DAVID, OUR FIRST CHILD

We returned to Baltimore and rented a second-floor apartment in the home of a relative of Shirley's on Piedmont Avenue. I returned to the Health Department. David was born at Sinai Hospital on the morning

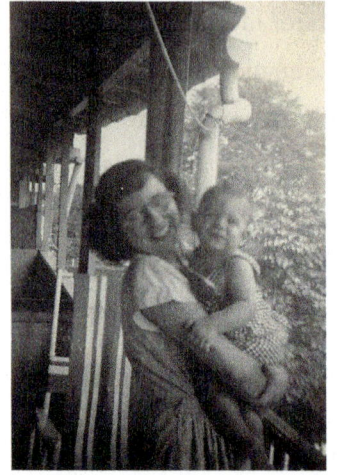

of December 15, 1947. I sat up overnight waiting for the birth. I went to work that morning, but made two stops on the way. I went to a barber shop and had a shave, the first and only time for a shave in a barber shop. I also stopped for several cigars which I distributed at work as I smoked one.

I recall dragging the heavy baby carriage up and down stairs to the second floor. There was a park with a lake not far from our apartment where we often took David. We had a back porch with stairs to the back yard. The ice man carried ice to our icebox through the back stairs. I took the street car to work.

During this period the director of

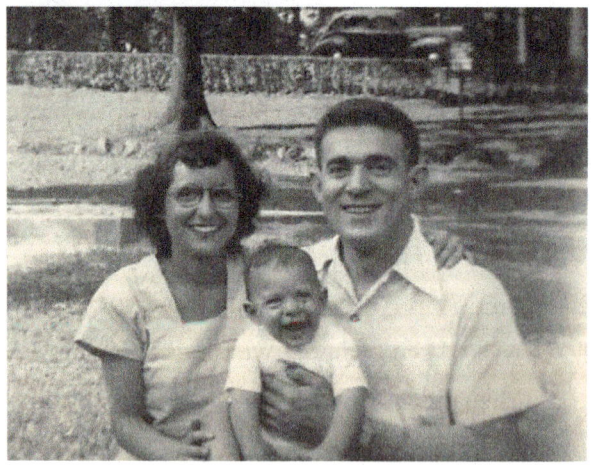

Top: David and Shirley. Above: David and his parents.

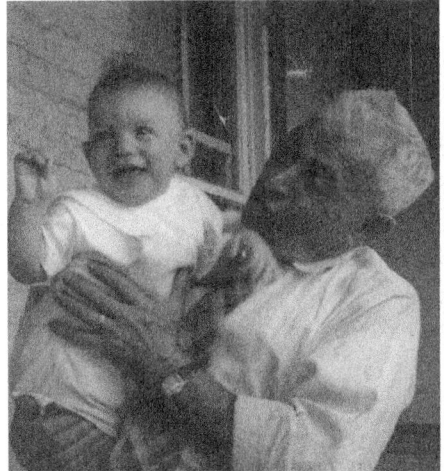
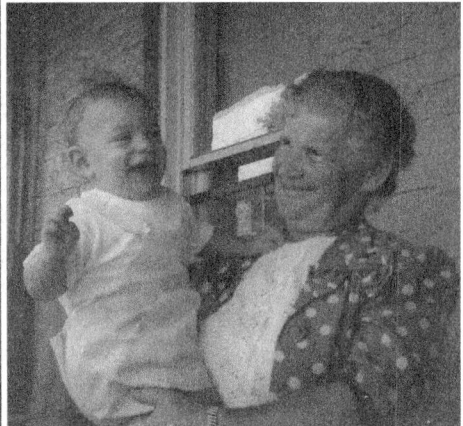

*Left: David and my father. Top right: David
and my mother. Right: A proud father.*

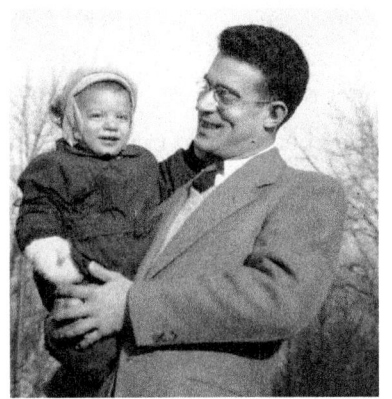

the Bureau of Heath Information in the
Health Department retired. Dr. Williams
had seen enough of my work that he
appointed me as director of that bureau.
I was responsible for issuing weekly
reports for the department designed to
get press coverage, editing the Monthly
Health News and the department's annual report.

I'M ON EARLY TELEVISION
1948

For years the Health Department had sponsored a weekly radio program.
It was now 1948 and television was beginning its appearance. Dr. Williams approached the television station owned by the *Baltimore Sun* and
asked for the department to sponsor a weekly education program. The
station agreed, and Dr. Williams and the Mayor announced the initiation
of the program, called *Your Family Doctor.* I played the part of the family
doctor, and named him Dr. Worthington after the first Health Commis-

Dr. Worthington on TV.

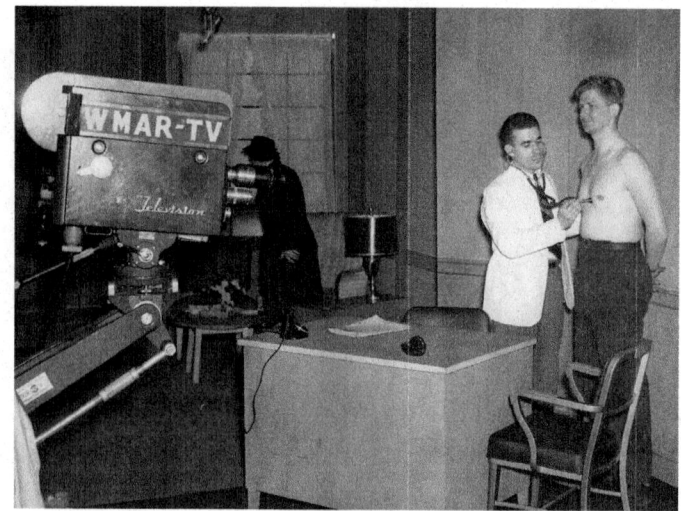

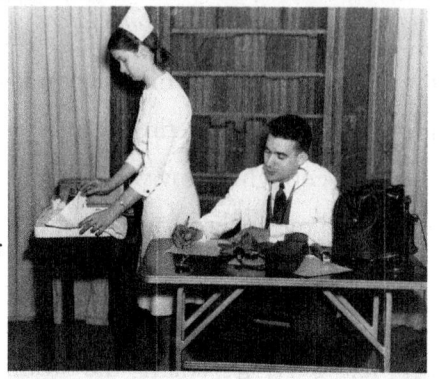

sioner of Baltimore. A nurse in the department played my nurse. I wrote the script each week, often about a communicable disease.

To assure the medical accuracy of the script, I submitted it each week to the director of the Bureau of Communicable Disease, Dr. J. Wilford Davis. We developed a close relationship. The nurse and I memorized our parts and performed live. At that time taping programs was not standard procedure, so we have no record except some of the scripts.

Shirley and I had a deep interest in the State of Israel. Her sister, Evelyn, married in 1948 and she and her husband Moshe Kerem moved to Israel and were among the founders of the Kibbutz Gesher Haziv. Shirley and I visited them in Israel several times. They had three children: Etan, Racheli, and Miriami. We attended Miriami's wedding. Racheli spent some time in the U.S. for graduate education. Evie, Moshe, and Etan have died. I keep in touch with Racheli.

ARAB-ISRAELI WARS

In 1947 in anticipation of the British plan to end their mandate over Palestine, the United Nations adopted the Partition Plan for Palestine, providing for a portion to be ruled by the Arabs and a portion by the Jews. In 1948 Britain ended its mandate. The Jews accepted the U.N. plan, but the Arabs refused. The Jews declared their independence and established the State of Israel. The Arab countries attacked, and a war ensued for six months. The Israelis were successful, and in 1949 an armistice agreement was signed by Israel, Egypt, Lebanon, and Syria. The boundaries were described as the Green Line.

In 1956 Egypt attempted to nationalize the Suez Canal, creating the Suez Crisis. Attacks on Egypt were mounted by Israel, Britain, and France. Israel captured the Sinai desert, but was forced to retreat.

In 1967 the Six-Day War took place. At-tacks on Israel were mounted by Egypt, Jordan, Syria, Saudi Arabia, Kuwait, and Algeria. The Israelis were victorious in six days. Israel captured the West Bank, East Jerusalem, and the Gaza Strip. The Israelis occupied these territories, lead-ing to unrest over many years. Peace efforts

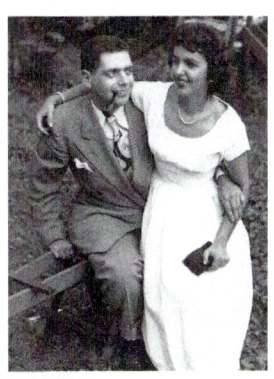

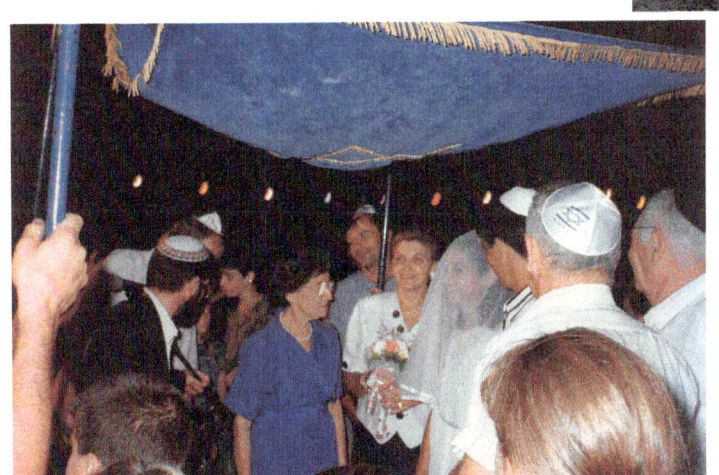

Above: Evie and Murray.

Left: We attend Miri-ame's wedding in Israel.

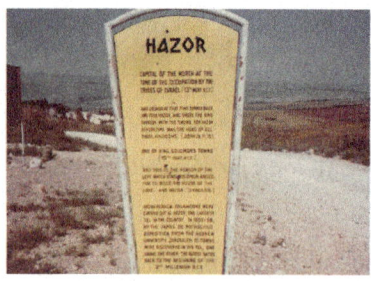

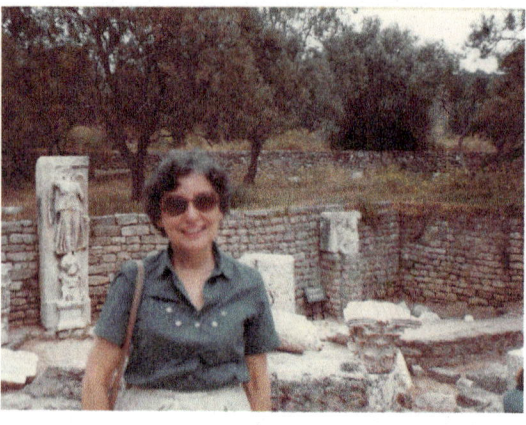

*Above: An ancient Israeli city.
Right: Shirley in an archaeological site in Israel.*

have failed to secure a resolution.

In 1973 Egypt and Syria attacked Israel on Yom Kippur. The Israelis defeated the Arab countries.

In 1982 the Israeli army invaded Lebanon to expel the PLO.

In 1987 to 1993 the First Intifada took place. The Second Intifada occurred from 2000 to 2005.

Shirley and I visited Israel several more times. Our interest in Israel has been deep and abiding.

WASHINGTON CALLED
1949 (I WAS 33)

*Left Shirley at the Israeli Memorial to President Kennedy.
Right: Moshe and Evie in an archaeological site in Israel.*

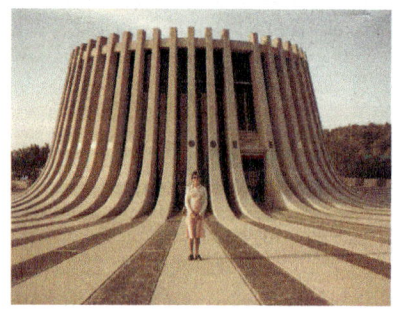

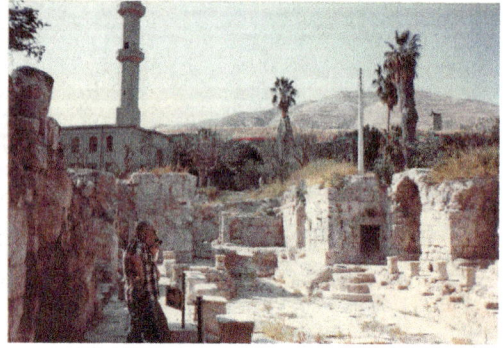

I was sitting at my desk at the Health Department one day when I received a phone call from Washington. It was a man named Arthur Kruse who was executive director of United Community Services of Washington. He described his organization, recently established as the successor to the Council of Social Agencies, affiliated with the Community Chest of Washington. Its mission was planning for improved community services for health, welfare, and recreation. It also was responsible for distributing funds raised by the Community Chest of Washington to the member agencies.

He was seeking a staff person as secretary of the health section of the agency and invited me to confer with him about the position. I agreed to meet with him, not without some trepidation, since this community task would be new for me. I took the train to Washington, and we had lunch in a hotel near his office. The offer was appealing, challenging. He impressed me as a person. I discussed the idea with Shirley and we agreed to make the change. (Later I learned how he reached me; he called the School of Public Health at Michigan and asked about recent graduates who had done well.)

We moved to Silver Spring, Maryland. Shirley had become friendly with a woman who had been a nursery school teacher in the co-op nursery school that David attended, and who also was a realtor. She suggested a small house at 622 Ray Drive in Silver Spring, which we purchased for $12,500, for which we obtained a mortgage. My office was in downtown Washington, at 1101 M Street, N.W. I took a bus to work, until one day Will arrived from Oklahoma City driving an old Dodge with a plastic roof. He was donating this car to us since he had several cars. We became friendly with a couple named Shapiro who lived two blocks away and had a daughter about David's age. There was also a couple with a young daughter around the corner with whom David played in our back yard. In fact, our yards adjoined, so we cut a gate in our fence to allow them to

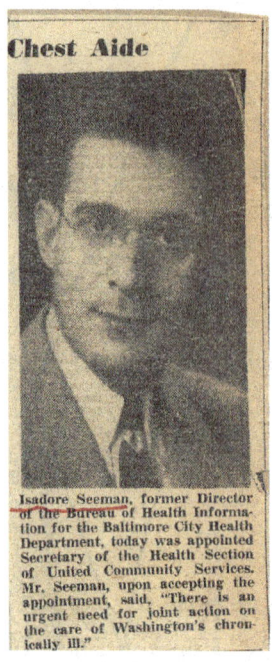

Chest Aide

My appointment to UCS.

get together easily. Shirley enrolled David in the Silver Spring Nursery School, a co-op program where she volunteered a day a week.

The Health Section of UCS had an Executive Committee which guided its work. The chairman of the committee was Dr. Winfred Overholser, the head of St. Elizabeth's Hospital, a federal facility for the mentally ill. I recall visiting him at the hospital located on very extensive grounds in southeast Washington, in his plush office. I also recall my first visit to another member of my Executive Committee, the head of Division II in the District of Columbia public schools, the segregated Negro schools in the city. I went to work on my new duties. I did an analysis of the major health issues in the city and obtained approval from the committee to undertake a study of nursing homes in the city. The number of such homes was relatively small, so I decided to visit each myself and complete a questionnaire. I carried this project out, exposing very poor accommodations and small staffs for very ill patients. I prepared a report which we publicized and received good press coverage.

We were eager to develop good working relationships with the D.C. Health Department. Just about the time I started work, the Director of Health, Dr. Ruhland, was retiring. I recall attending the retirement party for him together with my boss, Arthur Kruse. Arthur drove to his home in Northern Virginia after work and before the party. He offered me a drink. I had a martini. We drank a second before we set out. At the party I had another. I believe I came closer to being drunk than at any other time in my life. Dr. Seckinger succeeded him as Health Director, and I spent time developing relationships with him and key members of the staff of the Department. I remember developing close relationships with the head of child health, Dr. Ella Oppenheimer. One of the members of the Executive Committee was Dr. Paul Cornely, a professor of Public Health at Howard University. We developed a friendship that lasted many years. He was organizing the Washington Public Health Association to become an affiliate of the American Public Health Association, and I became a co-founder.

Most of the voluntary health agencies were not members of the Community Chest, raising money on their own: the Tuberculosis Association, the Cancer Society, the Heart Association, etc. Nevertheless, Kruse and I spent much time trying to develop relationships with these agencies.

Early in my assignment an issue arose which I tried to resolve. One of our member agencies was the Washington Hearing Society. This agency provided hearing tests free or at reduced fees to low-income persons, and recommended hearing aids for its patients. The private companies selling hearing aids objected to this practice that

In January 1953 Dwight D. Eisenhower was inaugurated as president of the United States.

impinged on their business. I undertook the task of trying to resolve the issue. I recall visiting the hearing section of Walter Reed Hospital Annex located in Silver Spring to enlist their counsel and aid. We were able to work out an acceptable agreement.

What happened in the 1950s?
The peace treaty with Japan was signed.
The Korean conflict took place.
McCarthyism engrossed the United States
The Brown vs. Board of Education Supreme Court decision
called for an end to school segregation.
President Eisenhower sent troops to Little Rock to enforce desegregation.
The Montgomery bus boycott was started.
DNA was discovered.

The first section of the Capital Beltway was opened.
Joseph Stalin died.
A Surgeon General's report announced that smoking caused cancer.
Rosa Parks refused to give up her bus seat.
Sputnik was launched.

Shirley and I became friendly with the couples who were also members of the staff of UCS, the Kruses, our deputy director and budget director, Ferdinand Grayson, the head of the welfare section, Paul Cherney, the head of volunteer services, Hulda Hubbell, and others. We visited them in their large Northern Virginia homes. I was especially close to Arthur Kruse and Ferd Grayson.

After several years Arthur Kruse decided to leave UCS and become head of the Community Chest of Chicago. Our deputy executive, Ferd Grayson, was appointed to head UCS, and he selected me to serve as Deputy Director and Budget Director. This broadened my responsibilities and gave me a wider perspective on all of the agencies in the Community Chest.

JONATHAN ARRIVES

In 1951 Jonathan was born at the Hospital for Women in Washington, D.C. Since David was only four years old, we needed to arrange for someone to stay with him when I drove Shirley to the hospital that night. Our friend Ruth Shapiro agreed to come and be with David. I recall that labor did not begin when we arrived, so the two of us watched a movie on television. The obstetrician advised me that delivery would be delayed, and I should leave the hospital for a few hours. I did so, driving around. I had left the house quickly and forgot to take any money with me. I hoped to get a cup of coffee while driving around, and I went to several gas stations hoping to use a credit card but get a few dollars in cash. I was unsuccessful and never got the coffee.

The house was small, with two bedrooms on the first floor. There was a finished attic on the second floor, one large room, with a low ceiling. We set this room up for the new baby. We registered Jonathan's birth giving him the name Robert Jonathan. Soon after we decided to switch the names and named him Jonathan Robert.

One day while still living on Ray Drive, Shirley received a call from New York informing her that her brother, Irvin, had died. The call was from a friend who had gone to Irvin's apartment and found him dead. Irvin was on the faculty at the Massachusetts Institute of Technology, but was on a one-year leave at Columbia University in New York. Shirley and I went to New York and to Irvin's apartment. We found empty bottles of sleeping pills. We also found a very recent letter from a girl discussing her break-off of relations with Irvin. It was clear he had ended his life in suicide. We knew he had had a troubled life, especially in relationships with women. I was required to go to the morgue to identify him. We then arranged to ship the body to Baltimore for the burial. We informed Shirley's father that Irvin had died of a heart attack.

MOVING TO DAMERON DRIVE

We felt that the house was now too small, and our income sufficient to allow us to move to a larger house. Shirley spent much time scouting the area looking for a suitable house. She found a house still under construction, a part of five similar houses that backed up onto Sligo Creek Park. We decided on this move to Dameron Drive to a one-story three-bedroom house with a ground-level finished basement with a recreation room and a fourth bedroom and a bathroom. There was no street in front of the house yet; we watched as they paved the street, but even then it did not go all the way to Forest Glen Road until a year later. Forest Grove elementary school, with a recreation area, was on the same street just three blocks from our house. We became very friendly with the owners of the other new four houses on the block.

David developed an abiding interest in baseball at a very early age. A memorable experience was his discovery of a card and dice baseball game called the APBA Game. He and Jonny spent hours on end playing the APBA game. The game involved shaking dice in a small cup with a metal bottom. The boys would awake early and begin playing the game. In order not to awaken the adults, they placed cotton in the bottom of the cup to deaden the sound.

THE VIETNAM WAR

In November of 1955 a civil war began between North and South Vietnam, later also involving Laos and Cambodia. North Vietnam was under communist rule, allied with China, and South Vietnam was independent, supported by the U.S. The U.S. interest was based on the view that a communist takeover of South Vietnam would spread broadly; the U.S. followed a policy of containment.

The U.S. first sent military advisors to South Vietnam. Later troops entered; troop levels tripled in 1961 and tripled again in 1962. Combat units were deployed in 1965. In all 2.5 million U.S. troops served in the Vietnam War. Presidents Kennedy, Johnson, and Nixon were all involved in decisions on the war. It was the war that caused President Johnson not to seek a second term. Neither side was able to win. U.S. military involvement ended in 1973. A Paris Peace accord was signed but was not effective in stopping the fighting.

In 1964 popular demonstrations against the war began. They involved civil rights groups, antinuclear war advocates, and college and graduate students. Demonstrations were held on campuses; 2,500 men burned their draft cards. Martin Luther King, Jr. participated in the anti-war movement. Shirley and I marched in several demonstrations. I recall one particularly cold day of one of the demonstrations; on leaving the demonstration, we were so uncomfortable that we stopped for a hot drink.

In August 1973 the Case–Church amendment was adopted ending U.S. participation. Later North and South Vietnam were united.

It was estimated that one million to three million Vietnamese soldiers and civilians were killed; 200,000 to 300,000 Cambodians; and up to 200,000 Laotians. U.S. military deaths totaled 58,200.

The Vietnam Veterans Memorial was built on the Mall in 1984. In 1995 President Clinton normalized U.S. diplomatic relations with Vietnam.

PHILIP ARRIVES
1958

In 1958, six years after Jonny was born, we had our third son. Philip was born at George Washington University Hospital in D.C. I remember our carrying him into the house. With a six-year gap between the youngest and a ten-year gap between David and Philip, the "older" boys treated Philip like a different generation. They played with him as their baby; they called him "the smartest baby in the world"; they sat on the floor and played with him.

An experience that would have important consequences years later was Shirley's acquaintance with the wife of a young couple who moved into the house on the corner across the street from us. They were Dr. David Willner, his wife Marilyn, and their newborn son, Shepard. David was a surgeon stationed at Walter Reed Hospital. Marilyn was the new mother of a newborn in a new neighborhood. She was lonely, and when she observed a stroller on our porch,

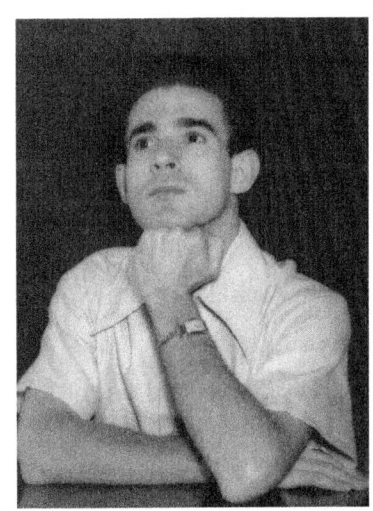

The younger Isadore.

she approached Shirley and asked if they could walk together with their babies. Shirley readily agreed, since she, too, was lonely with the older children in school. They became good friends. A few years later Marilyn had a second child, and since their house was small, they moved several blocks away. The mothers maintained contact with each other, even when the Willners later moved out of the state. This relationship had a major influence on my life many years later, as will be described.

Shirley's father moved from the original room we had rented for him to a second and then a third home which kept kosher and had a room to rent, providing meals. It was obviously a very lonely life for him, but there was no better alternative. We visited him in Baltimore, taking the boys along for a very dull afternoon. They usually played step ball while Shirley and I visited her father, with little to talk about. His health was not good, with heart disease and pulmonary issues. He developed pneumonia, was hospitalized for several days, and died in the hospital.

I Become the Executive Director of UCS
1954-1957

United Community Services was very closely affiliated with the Community Chest of Washington. Because fund-raising in the area depended in large part on solicitation from employees of the federal government and from major companies which extended beyond the D.C. boundaries, the six Community Chests had developed an organization known as the Chest Federation. It brought together on an informal, cooperative basis the separate Community Chests in D.C., nearby counties in Maryland, and counties in Northern Virginia.

UCS depended on the Chest Federation for our support, and we allocated most of the funds raised by the Chest Federation in D.C. to member agencies. A few years after I was named Deputy Executive Director of UCS, the head of the Chest Federation, Ed Keyes, retired. My boss, Ferd

Grayson, was selected to succeed him, leaving open the position of Executive Director of UCS.

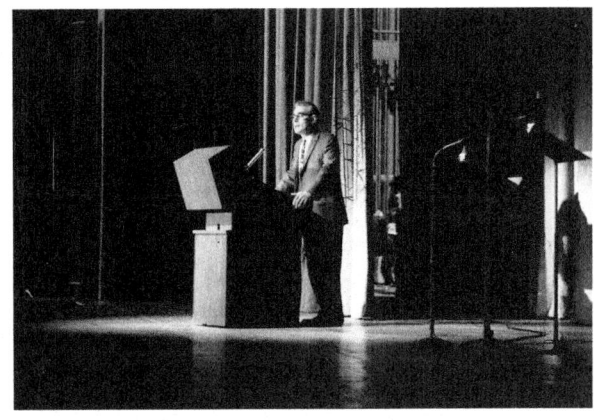

The leader of health and welfare services in the National Captial Area.

Clearly I was interested in moving up to this position. I applied, as did Paul Cherney, the secretary of the welfare section of UCS, and oth-ers. A personnel committee was appointed to select the executive. The chairman of this Committee was John Duncan, a member of the Board of Directors of UCS. John was one of the most important and effective members of the black community in Washington. He served as the Recorder of Deeds of D.C., the highest position in the D.C. government achieved by an African American up to that time.

I was interviewed by John as were the other applicants. Across the country the executives of organizations similar to UCS were typically out of the social work field, not public health. Typically, also, they were not Jewish. I recall in the interview with John I asked him if my being Jewish would have any bearing on the selection of the executive. John's reply: if you were black it would make a difference. I was appointed to the position.

What happened in the 1960s?

An American U-2 spy plane was shot down over Russia.
Adolph Eichmann was captured, tried in Israel, and executed.
Black students staged a sit-in in Greensboro, S.C.
The Bay of Pigs episode took place.
The Peace Corps was formed.
John Glenn was the first American to orbit the earth.

Rachel Carson published Silent Spring.
Martin Luther King, Jr. led the March on Washington, and made the "I Have a Dream" speech. My deputy, Tom Fetzer, and I joined the march and heard the speech.
Medicare was enacted.
Street cars stopped running in Washington
A peak of 543,000 U.S. troops was in Vietnam.
Thurgood Marshall became the first Black person to serve on the Supreme Court
John F. Kennedy, Robert Kennedy, and Martin Luther King, Jr. were assassinated.
Neil Armstrong became the first person to walk on the moon.

AN 18-YEAR PERSPECTIVE
1954-1972

I served for 18 years as the executive director of UCS and its successor agency, the Health and Welfare Council of the National Capital Area (more of that later). This was an exciting, rewarding, difficult, and challenging professional experience, and I devoted my best efforts to it. As a symbol of my determination to achieve effective results in the face of difficult obstacles, I treasured a statue of Sisyphus pushing a rock up the hill that held a prominent place on my desk.

Some specific experiences and aspects of those years are recited below, but it is important to understand the general nature of this responsibility and my position in it. These years were the most rewarding of my professional career. The agency I headed was responsible for disbursing up to $10 million annually to about 80 agencies from funds raised by the entire community. This gave me a unique stature in the community. I was invited to many community-wide meetings, often being asked to speak. The agency also developed working relationships with the local governments, especially on projects to improve community services in health and welfare. All of this occurred in a tumultuous period of moving from segregated services to integrated programming and attitudes. It was the active civil rights period. It was the period of the Vietnam War and its protests, and the period of John Kennedy and the social welfare initiatives of Lyndon Johnson's Great Society. I led the agency with a view to being actively engaged in these developments. I was responsible for appointing and supervising a staff of about 15 to 20 professionals. I led the agency to engage in several special projects. The agency was governed by a Board of Directors, many of whom were very important and prominent members of the business and professional community.

Among the community leaders who served on the Board or Committees of the agency were:

Katherine Graham, publisher of *The Washington Post*

Walter E. Washington, the first elected and the first black mayor of D.C.

John Hechinger, president of the large hardware chain in the area, and the first president of the D.C. City Council

John Duncan, the first African American to serve on the three-member D.C. Board of Commissioners

> *In January 1961 John F. Kennedy was inaugurated as president of the United States.*

W. Graham Claytor, Jr., a career diplomat and later the president of Amtrak

Alvin Steinberg, a wealthy owner of a debt collection company

William McManus, vice president of the Washington Gas Company

Robert (Rab) Wilson, vice president of the Potomac Electric Power Company

Ted Hagans, a wealthy African American, owner of a hotel serving primarily black persons and of several apartment houses, flying his own helicopter

Flaxie Pinkett, a prominent African American realtor

Mickey Bazelon, wife of a Judge of the U.S. Court of Appeals

Glenn E. Watts, president of the Communication Workers of
America

Lucille Maurer, Member, House of Delegates of Maryland

United Community Services
1954-1957 (I was 38)

Soon after I was appointed executive director of United Community Services, I was invited by John Duncan to his home. We met in his basement
recreation room, where there were eight or ten other African Americans.
As a leader of the black community, John had a corps of other blacks
monitoring and leading the civil rights activities in the Washington area.
We engaged in a conversation that was clearly aimed at making me aware
that my role in the movement was being watched. I had no difficulty in
assuring them that I would do all I could to further integration of community services.

Ferd Grayson had a brother-in-law in Ohio who was a Community
Chest worker. I brought Tom Fetzer to Washington to become my deputy, and Tom stayed with me for the rest of my service in Washington.
I also hired a new research director, Harold Goldblatt, whom I brought
down from New York City.

We had large committees of community volunteers who became
acquainted with the member agencies of UCS and made decisions about
which agencies could become members, and the annual allocation of
funds to each agency. We set standards for agency admission and worked
continuously to improve the quality of services. We administered a pay
scale for employees of UCS and the member agencies, and managed
agency participation in a national retirement plan.

CREATING A METROPOLITAN ORGANIZATION
1955-1957

I had a keen awareness that the District of Columbia and the nearby counties in Maryland and Virginia were one metropolitan community, interdependent. Many people crossed the borders daily for work, dining, entertainment, and other purposes. Some member agencies served the metropolitan region, such as the Boy Scouts and Girl Scouts, Catholic Charities, and others. To obtain their Community Chest funds, they were required to go to the separate Chests in each of the six jurisdictions. Each of the six Community Chests raised its own funds, but the annual campaign was coordinated by the Community Chest Federation, an informal arrangement to approach area-wide companies and the federal government personnel. I was determined to create a metropolitan-wide agency for planning and budgeting community services.

The process required careful planning, patience, flexibility, and diplomacy. I developed allies in the effort among the volunteer leadership, chief among whom was an attorney, Caesar (Jack) Aiello. It took two years to achieve the goal. I persuaded all six of the agencies to form the Inter-Chest Budget Group. This was an informal gathering of leaders from the six Chests to make recommendations on the level of funds to be allocated to each agency in the area. I also began working closely with the staffs in each Community Chest and Council.

We conferred with the lay leadership of each of the Chests and Councils, keeping the Chest Federation informed about our effort. It was very clear to me that we would not achieve a metropolitan-wide organization without developing a structure that retained functions in each of the six local jurisdictions. With this assurance that we would support a local planning function in each "region," we were able to obtain approval from all of the jurisdictions except the City of Alexandria. The executive of the Alexandria Council had a powerful voice among her lay leadership, and she would not give up her autonomy. To achieve our main goal, we agreed to bring Alexandria in on an informal basis. This arrangement lasted several years, after which the leadership in Alexandria saw that the other regions were satisfied, and Alexandria joined fully along with the others.

THE HEALTH AND WELFARE COUNCIL OF THE NATIONAL CAPITAL AREA (HWC) 1957-1972 (I WAS 41 TO 56)

I designed the structure of the new organization and drafted the Articles of Incorporation and bylaws and related documents with the help of attorneys on the Board. I recall traveling to each of the jurisdictions to obtain the signatures of the incorporators of the Health and Welfare Council of the National Capital Area. The new Board of Directors met and appointed me as Executive Director. The Community Chest of Washington, which had considerable endowment funds donated over the years, remained in existence but non-functioning.

About the same time that our movement to a metropolitan-wide organization was under way, one of the three commissioners of the District of Columbia, James McLaughlin, called a meeting of the county executives and Mayors of the suburban jurisdictions for informal discussions of common issues. This first informal step later led to the formation of regional committees, and later the formal organization of the Metropolitan Washington Council of Governments. I kept close touch with this movement, conferring with the staff person who headed the organizations as they evolved. Walter Scheiber was appointed executive director of COG, and I worked closely with him over the years.

The firmament for metropolitan-wide efforts reached in many directions. The Chest Federation had difficulty persuading the local Chests to give up their autonomy. The Federation took another direction. The lay leadership decided on establishing an organization that represented the givers, not the agencies that benefitted. The United Givers Fund was created. We now had sister metropolitan agencies for fund raising and for planning. The responsibility for allocation of funds to the agencies was retained by HWC.

From 1957 when HWC was formed to 1972 when I left HWC I provided leadership on many projects to improve health and welfare services in the region. I paid deliberate attention to programs in each of the jurisdictions by conferring with the lay leaders and the staff person in each of the jurisdictions, at the same time developing area-wide services under guidance by the metropolitan Board of Directors and Committees.

The work of monitoring the member agencies through lay committees and the membership and budget staff was an important function of HWC. In the process, we prepared standards and guidelines. At one point we issued the policy of requiring all agencies to provide services to persons of all races and ethnic backgrounds. Several agencies balked at the requirement, for example the Boys Clubs of Washington and the Florence Crittenden Home for unmarried expectant mothers. By persistent efforts, we achieved the goal.

In the process of reviewing agency functions and operations we closed several agencies. A home for African American seniors was providing very deficient services, and after failed efforts to improve, and with support from black leaders of HWC, we closed the agency. We reorganized the agency that was providing financial support to persons needing hospital care but ineligible for Medicaid and unable to pay the full cost. We simplified the process by assigning the function to the Hospital Council of the National Capital Area.

We developed studies and surveys of important issues, for example the need for day care for children of working mothers. Following evidence of the deficiencies in services, we organized the Child Day Care Association of the National Capital Area and provided initial funding to the agency. We conducted a study of the need for homemaker services for persons with disability, and organized the Homemaker Service of the National Capital Area. We had cooperation from the Visiting Nurses Association, and after debating whether it would be preferable to assign the new function to that agency, we decided that a separate agency would likely prove preferable. I provided the leadership in these efforts. These services continue today.

The District of Columbia operated an agency called Junior Village which cared for children who could no longer live with their parents. For years the quality of services was deficient and received publicity from the press about the harm to children. Katherine Graham, publisher of *The Washington Post*, took special interest in this issue. We organized a committee on child welfare services which led to a recommendation to close Junior Village and place the children in foster homes. Ms. Graham chaired this committee. The report of the committee contained a recommendation that improved children's services were needed at the neighborhood level. Out of this study we organized the Neighborhood Services Project with support from the Meyer Foundation which was established by *The Washington Post* family. We recruited a social worker from Chicago, Everett Cope, with good experience in neighborhood programs. He led the project with great imagination and effectiveness until he died from a brain tumor. Among the programs he instituted was the recruitment of residents of the neighborhood who had no professional training but who knew the neighborhood and would work with their neighbors to meet their health needs. When the project ended, the D.C. Health Department employed our neighborhood workers.

At one point I hired a new research director who suggested that we undertake a study of poverty in D.C. He knew of a prominent African American sociologist, Hylan Lewis, whom he proposed as director of the project. We succeeded in securing funds from the National Institute of Mental Health and undertook the project. Hylan was an imaginative leader. He employed an anthropologist who stood on street corners in a low-income neighborhood near our office and was successful in getting men in the neighborhood to talk with him, describing problems in their lives. Out of this aspect of the project the anthropologist published a book, *Tally's Corner.*

Hylan also employed a female social worker who received permission to live in a public housing project where she spoke with many women, listening to their stories of their lives. Out of this project she wrote a book, *Living Poor.*

When the project was completed, we received additional funds and employed a former newspaper reporter who led a project to publicize the results of the initial project. One of his accomplishments was to organize a public meeting on the project at which he secured Ossie Davis and Ruby Dee to enact some of the findings.

Through these projects we were able to provide documented information on the effects of poverty on the black community.

During this period the Urban Renewal Act was passed by Congress. It provided for acquiring and abolishing homes in poor neighborhoods and selling the land for redevelopment with public housing and low income housing as well as high income housing.

The D.C. Redevelopment Land Agency (RLA) was given responsibility for administering the program in Southwest D.C. I had worked with the head of the relocation service of RLA, James Banks. I designed a program to provide social services to persons required to leave their homes and move to a new neighborhood. RLA agreed to fund this project, and I employed staff to provide the services.

I worked closely with Jim during this project. We used a vacant residence in Southwest, in a house known as one of five Wheat Row houses constructed in the 1700s and destined to remain in the neighborhood. When the project was completed I hired a sociologist to review the program and write a critique.

There was a press account reporting on a story that the leaders in New Orleans were unhappy with the black community there, and were encouraging blacks to leave the city and move north. I recommended to the Board that HWC announce its readiness to receive any such persons and assure shelter for them. The Board adopted the resolution, but no blacks came.

In this period I attended many meetings with leaders of other planning organizations in the area: the National Capital Planning Commission which had responsibility for land use planning in the District, a group that worked on joint programs of educational institutions in the area, and others. I also became acquainted with an economist who was president of Resources for the Future, Harvey Perloff. Together we came to the conclusion that the region would be well served by a new planning organization which combined the functions of economic planning and coordinating the planning roles of the several planning agencies. We called it The United Planning Organization, (UPO). We recommended a Board of Directors including governmental and private representatives of the component agencies and lay community leaders. We were success-

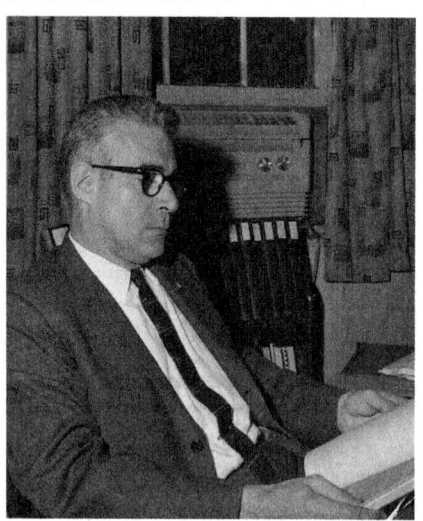

The studious executive.

ful in interesting the Ford Foundation in the project. Before the new venture got under way, an important development intervened.

It was at this time that Lyndon Johnson succeeded in getting Congress to pass the Economic Opportunity Act, beginning the War on Poverty. The act provided for a Community Action Agency to be established in each community to be funded by the act and to lead the anti-poverty effort. The structure of the Community Action Agency was essentially identical with the Board we envisioned for the United Planning Organization. It would have been conceivable to suggest that HWC become the community action agency for the region, but I determined not to pursue this effort, but instead to support UPO as the

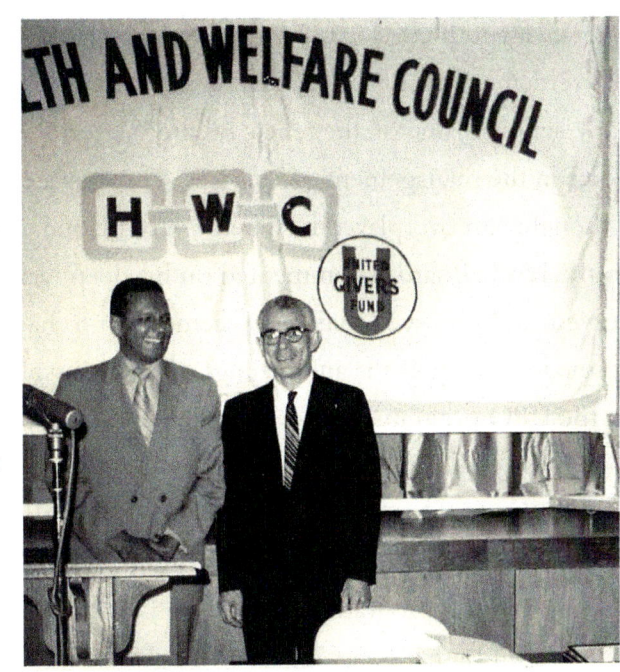

Above: Ted Hagans, president, and Sam Seeman, executive director, HWC.
Below: A rare invitation

antipoverty agency. In support of this goal, I had lunch with James Banks with whom I had worked before and urged him to become the executive director of UPO. He agreed. I also was in accord with the plan to select the former HWC president, Frederick Lee, to serve as president of UPO.

This was a tumultuous period for health and welfare services in the region. UPO had considerable funds to disburse, but chose its own course. HWC did receive funding to

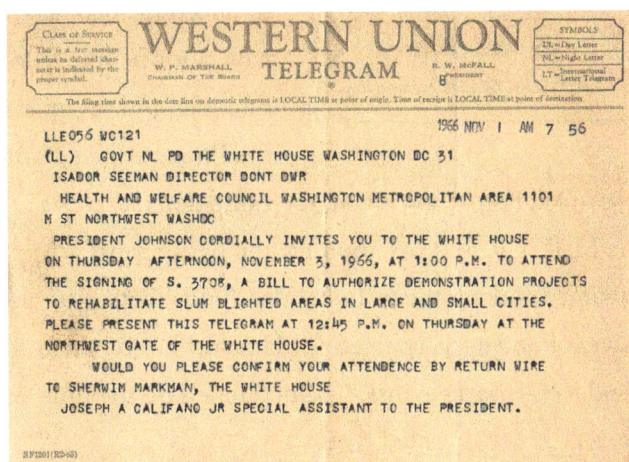

operate a youth employment program, which we administered through the settlement houses in the area. Under Jim Banks' leadership UPO took seriously one of the tenets of the War on Poverty, giving the poor a voice in the management of services. This was a commendable aim, but I thought Jim overplayed it. When Everett Cope died and I reported it to the HWC Board, I commented on his deep feeling for the people he served, and observed that UPO seemed not to have the same sensitivity to the individual needs and feelings of its clients. I said that I did not see in the UPO programs the love of people that Everett Cope felt deeply. The press picked up on this observation with a headline on page one of *The Washington Star.* It was probably due to this observation and publicity that I was asked to testify before a committee of Congress examining the War on Poverty program.

Martin Luther King, Jr., the civil rights advocate, was killed on April 4, 1968. Riots broke out in many cities, including the District of Columbia, with looting, fires and general turmoil. D.C. Mayor Walter Washington declared a curfew. One night as he planned to ride through the city to survey the damage, he invited me to join him in his car to help assess the destruction and the needs.

In November 1963, Lyndon B. Johnson succeeded to the presidency when John F. Kennedy was assassinated. Johnson was inaugurated in January 1964 after his own election.

Martin Luther King, Jr. had announced his plan to come to Washington with poor people from southern communities and set up a tent city as part of the Poor Peoples Campaign. Although he was killed before the event, the campaign did arrive and set up tents on the Mall. The issue of food for the participants arose, and HWC agreed to arrange food for them. I obtained funds from gifts and from the United Givers Fund and arranged for Howard University to prepare and deliver food to the participants. It rained much of the time and the site was a sea of mud when I visited there.

I MEET PRESIDENT JOHNSON
1966 (I WAS 50)

One of the programs that President Johnson proposed was the Model Cities Program. He enlisted aid from organizations to support the proposal. I was a member of the National Social Welfare Assembly with headquarters in New York and no office or staff in Washington. I agreed to represent the Assembly in meetings to support the program.

When the act was passed I was invited to the White House for the bill signing. There was a large gathering as the president signed the bill. After that each person came up to shake hands with the president. A military aide at his side asked my name as I approached the president. The aide whispered my name to the president, and the president called me by name as we shook hands. Later I was given a pen with President Johnson's name on it. About two weeks later I received a letter with a White House return address. In it was a photograph of me shaking hands with the president and a note saying, "The President

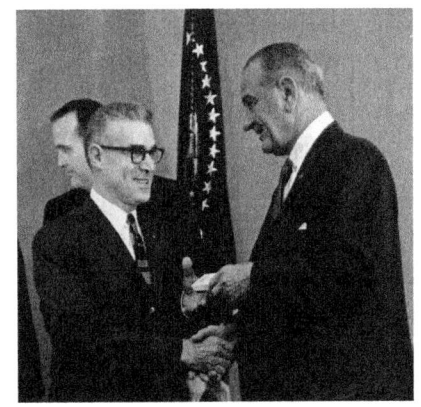

I meet President Johnson.

was looking at some photographs the other night and came across this photo which he thought you would like to have." Quite a memorable experience!

This was a period when President Johnson was successful in passing a great many new programs as part of the Great Society. I was invited by the Junior League of Richmond, Virginia to talk about these new programs. I had a meeting in New York a day before the Richmond event and flew up to New York. The next day, on the bus on the way back to the airport, I learned that there was a blackout. It was the blackout that affected the entire mid-Atlantic area. I arrived at the airport, but no planes were flying. I was due back in Richmond the next morning. How do I get there? I decided to take a bus back to the city, to the bus terminal. There were no planes and no trains. I took a bus to Washington, took a cab to the D.C. airport where my car was parked, and began the drive to Richmond. On the way I stopped at a service station and used the bathroom to shave. I made it to Richmond just in time for the talk. First I described my experience in the blackout, and I think that was as interesting to the audience as the talk on Great Society programs. A memorable experience!

Many of the meetings of the HWC Board were covered by the press, resulting in stories in *The Washington Post* and *The Washington Star*.

Annually I attended a conference of the executives of health and welfare councils across the country. We called ourselves the Million and Over Club, not for our salaries but for our community populations. I led the conference one year in Chicago.

Right: From the President.

THE WHITE HOUSE
WASHINGTON

Dear Mr. Sleemon,

The President was looking through some of his pictures today and thought you might like to have the enclosed.

Juanita D. Roberts
Personal Secretary
to the President

March, 1967.

The Family
1949-1956

With all of this professional work under way, I was still the husband and father of a young but growing family.

When David was still a baby, our first adventure with him was a trip to a state park in western Maryland. I recall stopping for lunch in a restaurant in Frederick on the way, where we took him in with a car-carrier and he was admired by all of the other patrons. We continued to take the children on vacations to state parks in western Maryland and to a state park in West Virginia, Cacapon State Park. There we slept in cabins with a fireplace burning wood. Each had a lake which we used for swimming. We walked on trails.

As the children grew a little older we took vacations in Ocean City, in Rehoboth, in Bethany, on Long Beach Island, and on Cape Cod. We stayed at the Finger Lakes in New York. Some of these vacations we took together with Ada Rhea, Shirley's sister, and her family: husband Ernie, and sons Ricky and Andy; Julie was not yet born. For several years I attended a social welfare conference at Silver Bay on Lake George in New York, and the children spent time in play groups organized by the conference; they were called the woozles, and the wee-woozles. One year I led the conference, discussing prevention in health and welfare services as the theme. Later the children attended teen camps in Massachusetts.

A 63-Year Marriage

This autobiography requires a section devoted to an analysis of the 63 years a husband and wife lived together. As background for this review, it is important to read a portion of a biography that Shirley wrote in 1963 about her early years and their lifelong influence.

"The tone of the home was gloomy and serious—an air of anxiety pervaded all our living. The family had a strange philosophy. They believed that we had to be content with less than others achieved for we somehow were not 'as good as' others. There were more important things than pleasures; namely, devotion to God and blind observance of religious ritual. My mother was the dominant parent although she was anything but a strong person. She was tense, anxious, very unsure of herself, with deep feelings of inadequacy. She cried easily, was given to pitying herself. She deprecated and criticized her children openly and extolled the virtues of other people's children.... My father was weak, colorless, ineffectual, irrational, and filled with fears and prejudices. He had little to do with the children but I remember being afraid of his ominous brooding silences, his unpredictability, and frequent and sudden quarrels with my mother."

"The dominant feeling about myself as a person during the years of my childhood and adolescence were those of unworthiness and inadequacy, and a strong conviction of physical unattractiveness.... I felt I could never please my mother or make her love me and the competition with the two unusually attractive younger children made it seem hopeless to try."

This background had a profound influence on my life with Shirley. There was never a doubt that we loved each other. We had many wonderful times together: at the theatre, concerts, dinners with friends, vacations, children's school experiences and growing up, Elderhostels, and other joyful times together. At a two-week Elderhostel in Venice it was

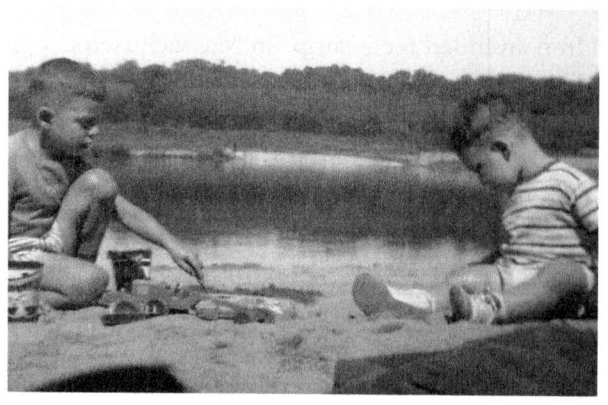

David and Jonny at Cacapon State Park, W.Va.

sheer joy and adventure. We took an auto trip to the Cabot Trail in Nova Scotia, Canada that was so enjoyable that when we returned I bought a wedding ring for myself which I had never had before.

At the same time, there was a tension that pervaded all too many occasions and experiences. We were, after all, two different people with different backgrounds, different early family experiences, different personalities. In many ways each of us hoped and sought to change the other to be more like ourselves, a fruitless effort. And there was Shirley's underlying depression growing out of her early family life. Her childhood left a lasting sense of lack of self-worth. Shirley was in therapy for most of her life. For the last 20 years she saw the same social worker weekly. Two of our children had problems that led us to seek therapy for them.

As a result, there

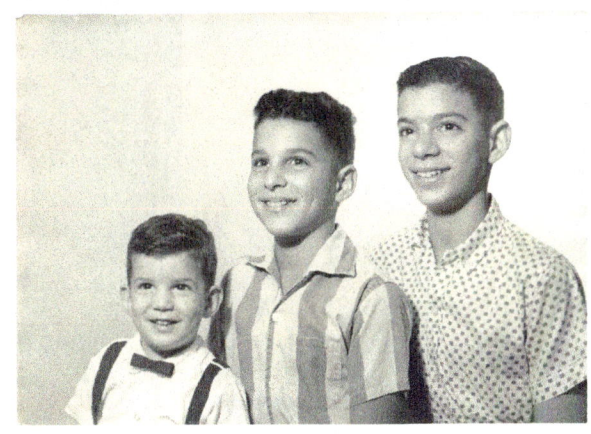

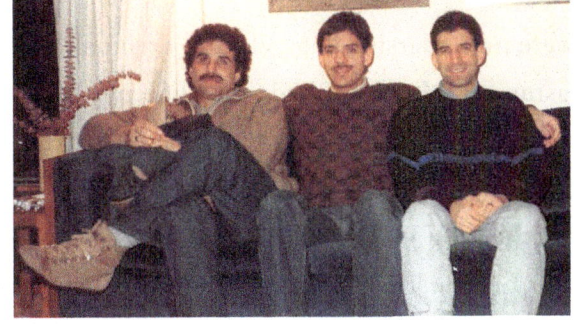

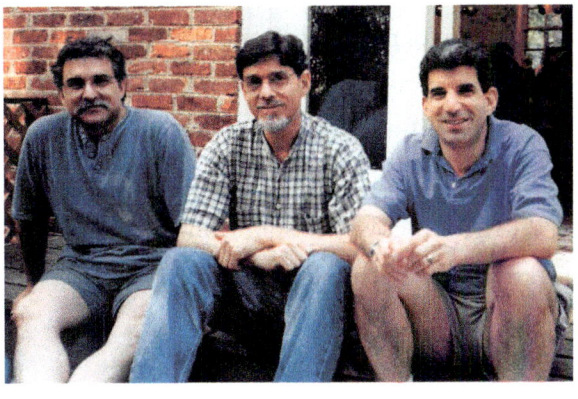

Top: Our three sons.
Middle: Growing older.
Bottom: Our grown sons.

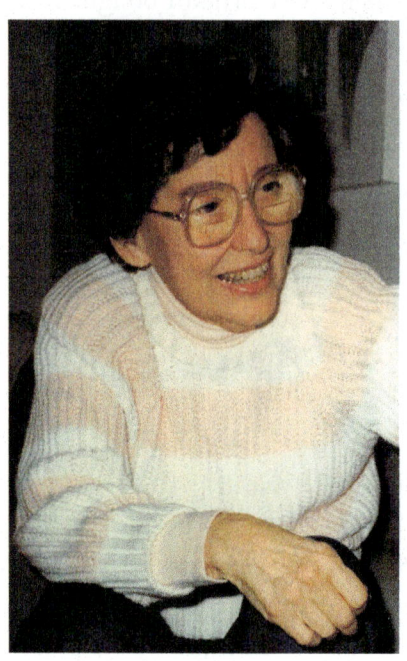 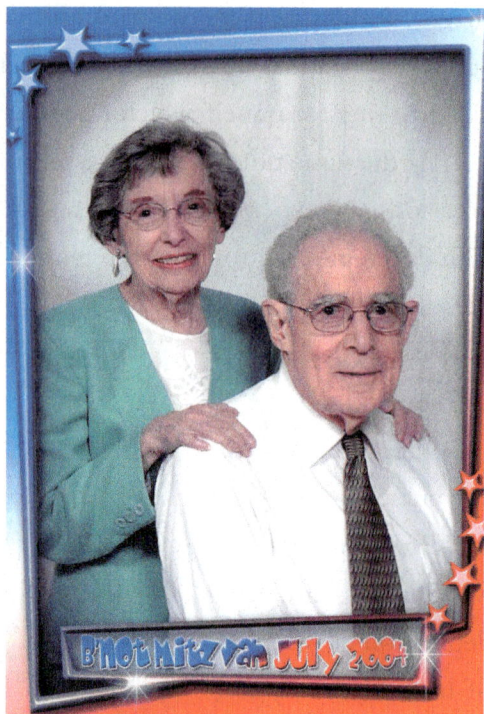

Left: Shirley admiring heer grandchild. Right: Shirley and me.

were misunderstandings, clashes, arguments, blaming, and my too-long-lasting withdrawals. I had great difficulty knowing how to respond to clashes. For a long time I took the view that it was Shirley's depression and behavior that was to blame, until one session we had together with the therapist made it clear to me that that approach was destructive, and that I needed to be aware that my own behavior needed to change and be more understanding and tolerant. I tried. On reflection now and with greater experience, I now understand a core problem in such relationships. Shirley would feel and express an anxiety, and I would offer her the solution. It was not a solution she was seeking; it was compassion, understanding, sensitivity, comfort and love.

I tried to comfort Shirley in rough times, not always with success. I wrote poems to her and for her.

Rendezvous

There is a shrine my soul
shall e'er revere,
A sacred wooded temple. In
That Place
My heart did burn so, time
can ne'er erase
The vision which my
memory holds so dear.
There did I speak of love to
her, so near
In heart, so near to me in close embrace.
Where better than by stream, calm current's chase
To carry off my each repressed tear.

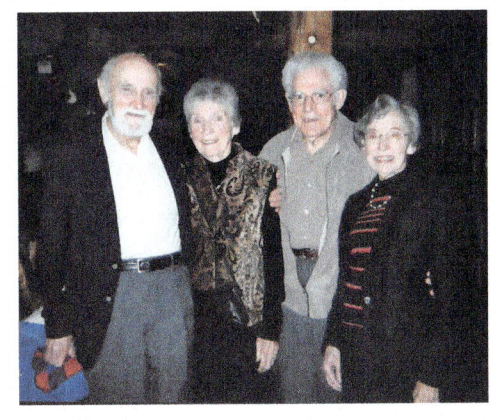

With Mef and Alice.

We rose aloft there as we sat that day
And talked of earth and sky, of God and man,
Stood high above where love alone holds sway,
In the dominion of "I dare, and can
Be what I will to be."— since I obey
The dictates of my heart, my head, and hand.

When the children were all in school, Shirley felt the need to return to professional work. She learned of a program sponsored by the National Institute of Mental Health which was designed to train women with no formal academic degree to become counselors to mothers of disturbed children. The program was operated by Children's Hospital in D.C. She applied and was accepted as one of eight students. She attended these classes for two years and graduated. She was then employed by the D.C. Department of Health and worked with mothers of disturbed children at D.C. General Hospital and at a nursery school in southeast D.C.

If You Dare Doubt

When swirling thoughts course swiftly through your mind
And leave confusion, wonderment, and doubt
In place of mind's peace, turn about
My love, and lead your thoughts to look behind
The veil of questions whose dark shadows blind
You to my everlasting love. From out
Of your abyss, my love divine shall rout
Each smallest demon, then draw forth and bind
Your soul but nearer to my heart than e'er
Before it dreamed. Ensuring peace, serene
As forest's majesty when tempests tear
Their futile forces through the unyielding scene,
Shall teach your heart---again it cannot dare
Doubt my eternal love, my heart's own queen.

One year when Philip was still in elementary school I served as president of the PTA of Forest Grove Elementary School. .

THE CHANGING FAMILY
1943

As I recall, I was the first of the Seeman boys to marry. Jules met Esther Millon at Teachers College, and they were married soon after my marriage. Jules had obtained his Ph. D. degree at Minnesota, then moved to Chicago where he worked with a prominent psychologist, Carl Rogers. I recall visiting him one year in Chicago. Later he moved to Nashville, Tennessee, taught and did research at Peabody College, later absorbed by Vanderbilt University. Jules had two sons, Larry and Bradley.

Mef met Alice Zerbola at Teachers College. He got his doctorate in sociology at Ohio State University, Alice got her Ph.D. in education, and they were married and moved to Malibu where he became professor at the UCLA. They had a daughter, Teresa, and a son, Paul.

Will got his Ph. D. in Minnesota. He found a teaching position in Oklahoma City, later worked at the Mayo Clinic, and then was appointed professor of psychology at the University of Cincinnati. He married quite late and had one son, Jeffrey. The marriage did not last and he was divorced. The Seeman family was now scattered across the country.

I organized several family reunions to keep us in touch with each other. All of my nieces and nephews attained professional careers. Will's son Jeffrey applied his computer skills at a book publishing company. He had a life-long devotion to the guitar and produced a professional album of nine original songs using the slide guitar. Gussie's son Harvey became a civil engineer in the transportation field. Her daughter Esther created and was CEO of an educational agency training active citizens to become better community leaders. Jules's son Larry followed his father as a psychologist, and Bradley applied his public relations skills for non-profit organizations. Mef's son Paul studied law and served as a judge in a juvenile court. His daughter Teresa was affiliated with the Medical School at UCLA and conducted extensive research on health services.

My father smoked two packs of Helmar Turkish cigarettes a day for most of his life. He also had several shots of whiskey every day, in spite of efforts by my mother to end the practice. My father complained regularly of lung problems. When the children were all grown and away from the house, my parents decided to move to Florida. They had limited means, but managed to purchase a house in Miami. Later they moved to an apartment in Miami Beach. I visited Florida with my family to see them each year for several years, always in the summer when I could get away from the office. Later my aunt Ruth moved to Florida to be near my mother, her sister. Ruth had taught Hebrew School in Scranton, PA for many years, visiting us every few years, always bringing presents for her

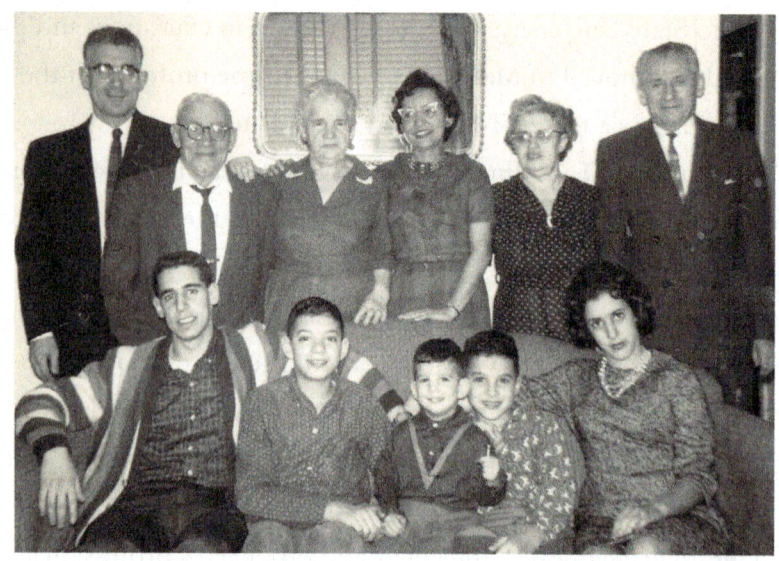

nephews and her niece. She married late, and when her husband died, she remarried and moved to Florida. My sister Gussie married somewhat late to Sol Berlin, a baker, and she had two children, Harvey and Esther, both of whom made very successful careers. When they were grown, she, too, moved to Florida to be near our parents.

While in Florida, Gussie found a copy of an autobiography that

Above: I organize a family reunion. Below: The family together.

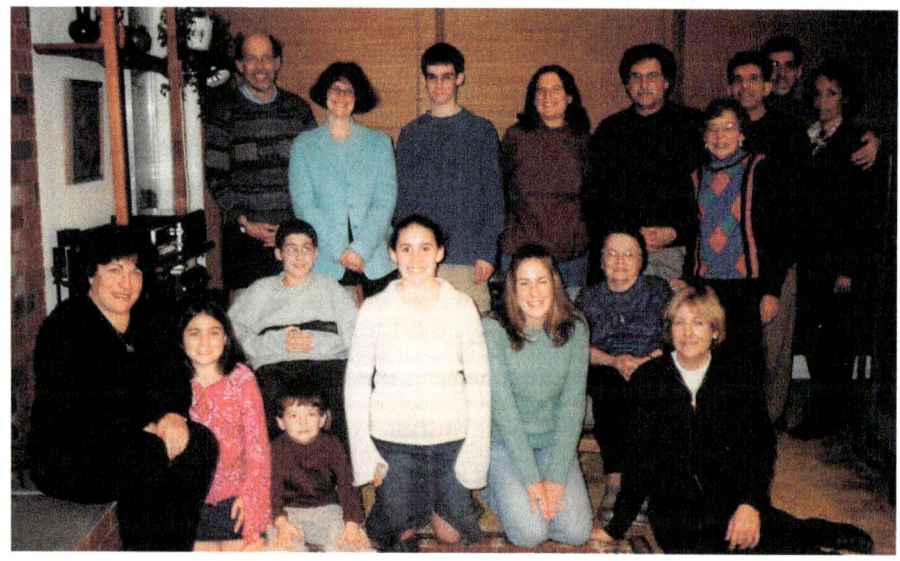

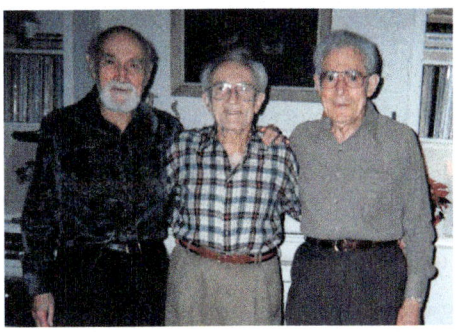 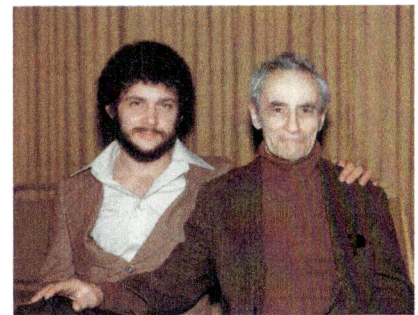

Left: The three remaining brothers. Right: Will and Jeffrey.

my mother wrote. It was all too brief. It was a very moving account, describing my father's courtship in Austria, her rejection of him at first, his courtship a second time after he returned from the army, and her reluctant agreement to marry. She was extremely unhappy in the marriage throughout her life and described it dramatically. in her autobiography, which I quoted from on page 14. My father was immature throughout his life, with no understanding of a loving relationship with a wife or with children. My mother did her best to try to hide this from the children, but this is the atmosphere in which we grew up.

I had a very troubling experience one day. My parents owned and rented out two "slum" houses in Baltimore, one of which contained a store front. Both were deteriorating and harder to rent. My mother called me one day and asked me to arrange to sell them at auction. I hired an auctioneer who advertised the sale. I went to Baltimore to the first house, where

> *In January 1969, Richard Nixon was inaugurated as president of the United States.*

about a dozen or more persons were present and bid on the house. The price agreed on was not very high, but I had to accept the highest bid. We then went to the second house with the store front. The auctioneer and I and one other person met there. With only one person present, there was no bidding. The one person offered a ridiculously low price, and the auctioneer advised me to take the bid, since we would need to hold another auction if I refused. I took the bid. A few minutes later all of the people who had been at the first house appeared. I was very troubled that the auctioneer should have known that the others would show up and bid. I complained, and wrote a letter to him later, but it was too late. When I informed my mother of the poor return on the houses, she did not complain, but I had a hard time falling asleep that night after the disaster of the auction.

Shirley and I were sitting at home one evening in 1963 when we received a phone call from Florida. It proved to be a great shock: my mother had died. The circumstances made it even more bizarre: she had bought two ice cream cones and was crossing the street to her apartment to share them with my father when she was struck by an automobile and died. Shirley and I hurried to Florida. The funeral service was impressive; she had been very active in the Pioneer Women's movement for Israel and a large crowd attended the service. She was buried in Miami. My father showed little sign of grief; his chief observation was about how many people attended the service. On the way to the cemetery I cried.

My father lived alone for a time until we arranged for him to live with a family where he could get his meals. His condition deteriorated; on our visits it was clear he was in early dementia. We moved him to a nursing home and the brothers shared the expense. He died in 1969 and he, too, was buried in Miami.

FAMILY FINANCES
1916-2011

Throughout my life my economic circumstances have ranged from genuine poverty to a comfortable and secure retirement. Except for the brief period when my parents owned the restaurant/whiskey business, the family income was insecure and borderline adequate until the boys went to work. I do not believe we ever received financial assistance, but there was the period of homelessness when we lived on the farm, and for many years my mother took in foster children to increase our income.

When Shirley and I married in 1942 I was earning $2,400 a year, then considered a fairly decent salary for a two-person family. Of course, Shirley was also working. In the early years of our marriage, with children adding to family expenses, and paying a mortgage, our family budget was tight. We regularly had to make a monthly decision on which bills to pay and which to defer until the next paycheck. To purchase our first house, we had to borrow for the down payment from my parents, who themselves had limited means. We borrowed from Will and my parents to finance our education in New York, even though I was working part-time.

My income increased when I moved to Washington, as did our expenses as well, but we were more comfortable financially. When I reached executive positions, income increased. In my later work for the government, salaries improved. We then began savings and investments. In the later years we had adequate income, though Shirley often had difficulty accepting the reality. We learned that many people who grew up during the depression had difficulty ever shaking the experience.

By the time of my retirement, with continuing contract work, our income provided security.

LOVE AND ANGUISH

Shirley and I never doubted our love for each other, yet there were times when our personalities and past experiences stood in the way of effective and compassionate communication.

The Trap

Life is a trap. We do no ask to come,
But screaming, we must exit from the womb

And enter this imponderable tomb,
This grand enigma, world we cannot plumb.

Nor can we choose the time when we must go.
Bound by the laws of nature and of chance,
We're doomed to play the play, to dance the dance.
Seek no escape. The trap has willed it so.

To stay is to be caught in deep travail,
To go is to negate what brought us here
And trade this earthly hell for hells to fear.
Between the two, we're trapped to moan and wail.

Turn right and there we find the way is barred
By walls and fences insurmountable.
About face, there incalculable,
By monsters and by dragons we'll be charred.

Climb up and up and at the top is found
Impenetrable barriers of stone.
Retreat, and down below, there all alone
Into a pool of blood we're surely drowned.

Move forward---see the fearful sight now loom
Before your eyes---the fires of hell on earth.
Flames leaping high, no lack, no dearth
Of red hot ashes certain to consume.

Retreat and face a greater enemy
Than all the torture physical---the pain

Of mental anguish. Know that they are vain,
Attempts to escape this mental slavery.

Why am I here? Why born into this life?
Who is to say the purpose of this game?
No man can fathom it, give it a name,
Except to know that it is Gethsemane.

Life is dilemma, two paths both bearing horns,
Between the two no passage, no wide gap
Through which we can escape this mortal trap.
"Surrender", comes the cry, "Give in" life warns.

Yes, there were periods of misunderstanding and distance between us. In time and with the help of Shirley's therapist whom we occasionally visited together, I realized how much I contributed to the difficulties. Then there were times of beautiful harmony and joy.

Testament to My Love

Deep have I sunk,
    And felt the very floor of endless hopelessness;
Thought to have dug
    My own mired pit of black despair,
Below the ken of suns
    That man must see to see
The light; beneath e'en hope
    Of hope to e'er return;
Then deeper yet, and deeper still
    Have borne my leaden soul,
Until the dread dark door
    Of very death, the final fall,

Seemed like the light,
And sole hope
Of once more being master,
    Or no more.
Then came my love with love,
And like to nothing
    That the earth or men upon it
May e'er know
    Or ever dream to know,
The love which she and I
    Have built with timbers of our souls
Did find me out
    E'en in my bottomless pit
And step by step, by small degrees,
    Did raise me up
To stature I once knew, and taller still
    Than e'er I hoped to be.
Here now do I stand
    Challenging the sun's own glory,
The radiance of heaven
    And, man's own joy,
Noble – bold testament to my love.

THE GREAT SOCIETY

After his election in 1964, President Lyndon Johnson determined to enact legislation aimed at eliminating poverty and promoting racial justice. These efforts were, in part, a follow-up to President Kennedy's New Frontier that was stalled in Congress.

Johnson had the advantage that in the 1964 election both houses of Congress had more than a two-thirds majority of Democrats. In addition Johnson's skill in enacting legislation was masterful. He created

14 task forces to design new programs, led by Bill Moyers, Presidential Assistant, and Richard N. Goodwin, his speechwriter. Johnson submitted 87 bills to Congress and 84 were enacted. In a speech written by Goodwin Johnson described the effort as The Great Society. Among the War on Poverty programs enacted were the following:

The Economic Opportunity Act

Community Action programs

The Job Corps

The Neighborhood Youth Corps

Medicare

Medicaid

The Older Americans Act

VISTA

The Model Cities program

Upward Bound

Food stamps

Head Start

The Elementary and Secondary Education Act

The Higher Education Act

Among the civil rights bills were the following:

The Civil Rights Act of 1964

The Civil Rights Act of 1965

The Civil Rights Act of 1968

Other programs included the following:

The National Endowment for the Arts and Humanities

The Corporation for Public Broadcasting

The John F. Kennedy Center for the Performing Arts

The Department of Transportation

The National Highway Traffic Safety Administration

The Omnibus Housing Act

Creation of the Department of Housing and Urban Development

The Air and Water Quality Act
The Wilderness Protection Act

AN UNCOMFORTABLE ABORTED MOVE
1969

There was a point in my work at HWC when I became somewhat rest-
less. I looked at some other possibilities. Then an opportunity became
available. HWC, as other health and welfare councils, was a member of
Community Chests and Councils of America. This organization provided
assistance to local agencies through annual conferences and staff guidance. I participated in these meetings and knew the staff.

The head of the planning staff informed me of a vacancy as the
health staff person and offered me the position. I gave it some thought
and was attracted to the idea of serving at the national level. I accepted,
but also had some misgivings about the travel aspects, especially with the
kids still at home. To help me deal with these reservations, I flew out to
Cleveland where my former boss, Arthur Kruse, was now living. Arthur
was very familiar with the field. I conferred with him, and he was definite
in discouraging me from taking the position. He not only commented
on the travel issue, but advised me that the organization did not take
the role of advice to local groups on planning very seriously or effectively. Its main focus was on the fund-raising role. Reluctantly, and with
much personal embarrassment, I called the head of the council program
and informed him that I was withdrawing from the position. I was very
troubled but felt I needed to drop out.

The *Washingtonian* magazine published a long article about the
United Givers Fund and the Health and Welfare Council. The article was
quite critical of UGF, on the basis of both its fund-raising and its record
on representation of blacks. In fact the UGF Board of Directors had
only one black person in its membership, whereas HWC was well repre-

sented by black members on the Board and committees. In part because of this poor representation of African Americans on the UGF Board, a separate Black United Fund had been established. Since HWC represented blacks in its operations and the member agencies, I saw no need for this separate black fund, but we had to live with it.

I Change Jobs
1972 (I was 56)

I served for 23 years in the Washington area with UCS and its successor HWC.

Then I did change jobs, but under different circumstances. Ferd Grayson left UGF and returned to his home in New Orleans. He was succeeded as head of UGF by Ralph Smith. I had to develop relationships with the new executive. It became clear to me that he did not have the competence for the job and was not open and straightforward. As time moved on several persons in his lay leadership began to hold the view that UGF raised the money and UGF should be the agency to allocate it to the member agencies. Such a move would seriously undermine the role of HWC. The planning function without funds behind it would be much less effective. I realized that I could not fight this move, since UGF had the funds and could make the change. I decided it was time to leave before this change occurred.

I resigned from HWC in September 1972, and a "Salute to Sam" luncheon was arranged. I received letters from several people who were unable to attend. Among them was a letter from the executive director of the National Children's Center. It read, in part:

"The community lost a most able leader and a man who demonstrated over and over his total commitment to the betterment of urban communities and was most influential in bringing about many badly needed services and in educating its citizenry in their brotherly responsibilities and communal commitments… We hope you will maintain the friendship of the leaders of the social service agencies who looked up to you with such respect."

An attorney wrote, "I suppose that many of us have taken you for granted and on reflection I now realize that it was because of your quiet manner and your objective approach to the rather difficult job of running the Health and Welfare Council of the National Capital Area. You have been a source of great strength during a most critical period and your contributions to the Washington community will be felt for many years in the future."

Msgr. Cody wrote: "May I express to you my own personal appreciation and that of all of us at Catholic Charities for your years of leadership at HWC. The problems that you faced were many and trying ones, but you were always able to bring to them a sense of balance and wise judgment."

Two years after I left, HWC no longer existed. The United Fund decided that it would take over the budgeting function that HWC had handled; HWC merged into the United Fund, and the planning function of HWC was essentially abandoned. Soon Oral Suer became the head of the United Fund. A few years later he went to prison for embezzling campaign funds.

Before resigning I began to look for other employment. One day Shirley saw a notice in *The Washington Post* that the U.S. Department of Health, Education and Welfare (HEW) was seeking a person to head the health branch of the budget office. I inquired and then applied for the position. I met the qualifications. I met with the head of the budget office and with his supervisors. They agreed to hire me, but it required some personnel maneuvering. On the list of eligible applicants for the position was a veteran who would take preference in employment, but he was not the person they wanted for the position. To arrange my appointment, rather than draw from the list for this position, they appointed me to a special position at the National Institutes of Health, with the understanding that I would then be transferred to the budget position as an inter-agency move. I signed in at NIH, and then signed the waiver to allow me to be transferred to the budget position.

This move gave me a whole new perspective. The position was held in high esteem by the heads of the health agencies in HEW because I could make recommendations that could seriously affect their appropriations. I met with the heads of each of the health agencies, including NIH, the Health Services and Mental Health Administration, (HSMHA), the Indian Health Service, the Food and Drug Administration, and others. I had a staff of three persons whom I supervised, and I reported to the head of the budget office. I learned a great deal about the many federal health programs.

An interesting event occurred very soon after my appointment. One of the tasks of the office was to prepare responses for the Secretary of HEW on incoming letters. A letter was sent to the Secretary from the head of the D.C. Mental Health Association, a person I had worked with in HWC, urging the Secretary to override the recommendation from the Office of Management and Budget (OMB) to cut funds for Community Mental Health Centers. This occurred when Richard Nixon was president and OMB had taken the position that it was time to cut funds for Community Mental Health Centers because they had proved they were successful and could now stand on their own. This was hardly a position I could support, but I was required to draft a reply that supported the OMB decision.

> *In August 1974, Gerald Ford succeeded to the presidency when Richard Nixon resigned. Ford was inaugurated in January 1977 after his election.*

The budget process involved recommendations from the Secretary that were sent to OMB. OMB then prepared their decisions on what could be sent to Congress. I recall my first encounter at OMB. It was on Christ-

mas day, and I went to their office and was given "the mark," the level of
funding they decided on for each health program. These recommendations
were then used in the HEW submission to Congress. I accompanied the
head of the budget office when we were called to testify before the health
subcommittee of the House Ways and Means Committee.

One day a memo crossed my desk requesting the opinion of the
budget office on a proposed new procedure regarding the Hill-Burton
Act. I wrote a serious reply, but my inclination to rhyme and whimsy was
tested. I also sent the following memo to my superiors.

The Ballad of Title VI

February 5, 1973

NOTE FOR : MR FORBUSH
MR. MILLER
MR. CARDWELL

*SUBJECT; Comment on Proposal for Direct Loan Procedures in
the Hill-Burton Program (or The Ballad of Title VI.)*

Those Congressional peers, Hill and Burton,
Said our hospital system was hurtin',
They wrote up a bill
Granting millions, until
The need for more beds was less certain.

Then we turned to a system of loans,
Adding subsidy to cushion the groans.
We buy and sell bonds
As the market responds.
Now we have to keep up with Dow Jones.

Meanwhile, back at Parklawn,
The financiers were working 'till dawn,
Devising a caper
To market the paper.
Attached is the plan that they've drawn.

To concur or not to concur,
That is the question, dear sir.
Do we add our consent
To the memo we're sent?
It's an issue we cannot defer.

While the position's before AS/C,
Across town is heard a decree.
There's no doubt of the source,
It is coming, of course,
From the oracle called OMB.

They've made perfectly clear their desire,
Section 626 must expire.
It all ends, you recall,
Loans, grants, and all,
When the mortgages written retire.

The securities now in our hand
Must be offered for bid throughout the land.
Though we tried Fannie Mae
It won't do, so they say,
We must peddle them as our own brand.

So let's set up the system proposed,
Though just after it's opened, it's closed.
   If we fail to do it
   By GAO we'll rue it.
There's no point in being opposed.

This analysis may lack precision
Except for one major decision.
   This rings down the curtain
   On dear old Hill-Burton.
It will soon be only a vision.

During my tenure in this position I developed relationships with other offices in HEW, including the office of Planning and Evaluation. After about two years, I found the budget position to involve a great many routine tasks and that there was limited opportunity to have real effect on decisions. However, my performance on the job was observed by the head of the health division in the Office of Planning and Evaluation, and he invited me to join his staff. This opportunity appealed to me and I accepted. I was assigned to head the Evaluation Unit in the office.

I found this position challenging. Congress had enacted a provision that set aside one percent of each appropriation to a health program to be used to evaluate the program. Based on this law, our office required each agency to submit to us a plan for evaluating its services. I supervised this effort. I met with the staff person in each of the agencies who was in charge of evaluation. As this process proceeded it became clear to me that there was not an effective system for carrying out this program. I held many meetings with the responsible staff, and out of that I drafted an improved procedure. I submitted this plan to my boss, who in turn submitted it to the Assistant Secretary for Planning and Evaluation and the Assistant Secretary for Health. Both approved the plan with commendations on its preparation.

During this period the Office of Planning and Evaluation was heavily involved in drafting a proposal supported by President Nixon for a national health insurance program. It was actually a generally liberal program. I observed and made occasional comments in the drafting, but was not directly involved. The bill was submitted to Congress but never adopted.

As time moved on, the next election took place and Jimmy Carter was elected. This meant that my boss and others who were Republican political appointees would leave the administration and be succeeded by Carter appointees. That left me as the senior person in the health branch of the Office of Planning and Evaluation. Before he left, the Assistant Secretary for Planning and Evaluation appointed me as Acting Deputy Assistant Secretary for Health Planning and Evaluation, a distinguished position indeed.

That role lasted for several months until the Carter appointee arrived, Karen Davis. I worked under her for several years. She was heavily involved in drafting a Hospital Cost Containment Bill for submission to Congress to deal with the high cost of health and hospital care. I participated; I accompanied her in testimony to Congress and made trips to speak to hospital groups in Vermont and Nashville. The bill was never adopted.

Once again my work was observed by another unit in what was now called Health and Human Services—the Office of the Assistant Secretary for Health. Dr. Julius Richmond was the Assistant Secretary and the Surgeon General of the Public Health Service. He was the author of the Head Start program in the War on Poverty. One of his deputies invited me to join that staff. That appealed to me, and I made the move. I was named chief of the Planning and Research Branch, and had the opportunity to work closely with Dr. Richmond. Two assignments were particularly memorable. The authorization for the department's program to

In January 1977, Jimmy Carter was inaugurated as president of the United States.

recruit and train health manpower was expiring, and its renewal was being drafted. When the bill was ready for submission to Congress, Dr. Richmond was preparing to testify for it. I undertook the task of drafting his testimony, and he was very pleased with the result. At another point Dr. Richmond was eager to propose a program to deal more effectively with the problem of infant mortality. I was assigned to draft a proposal. I brought together representatives of the all of the units in the department concerned with this issue. Reaching agreement on a unified plan was not easy. I told the group I would lock the door until we came up with a viable proposal. We did so, but it was never enacted.

ANOTHER JOB CHANGE
1980 (I WAS 64)

A change occurred in my direct supervisor in the office of the Assistant Secretary for Health. A woman who was very rigid in her views about how to deal with staff, and not at all friendly, was assigned. I did not get along well with her. For example, when I completed the report of the infant mortality project, she insisted that I rewrite the report into a format she had designed, whereas I had prepared the report that I thought conveyed its purpose adequately. I refused to comply, and she complained. I took the issue to Dr. Richmond and he upheld my view. But I remained uncomfortable under her supervision.

The person who had recruited me to this position was aware of my discomfort, and she arranged a transfer for me. I was assigned as director of the Division of Evaluation in the National Center for Health Services Research. This position gave me new perspective on the field of health services research. One of my tasks was to prepare brief summaries of completed research for publication in our newsletter.

I was in this position for about two years when Congress expressed its unhappiness with the work of the center, and in particular with the director and the assistant director. They cut the budget and staff severely, and my position was eliminated. I could have been terminated from federal employment, but again my relationships with others in the department came to the rescue. The director of the National Center for Health Statistics (NCHS), Dorothy Rice, had observed my work. She arranged for my transfer to her office. I was assigned to the Division of Planning and Analysis, but with no clear assignment. Soon

> *In January 1981, Ronald Reagan was inaugurated as president of the United States.*

after, she called me into her office and asked if I would like to undertake the task of manager of a new survey she wished to be launched. It was a National Mortality Followback Survey. The office had conducted four such surveys, but none for the last 18 years. I readily agreed and found the next two years exciting.

The survey involved designing and executing a questionnaire mailed to the next of kin of a national sample of persons who had died the previous year. I was assigned to the Mortality Statistics Branch, with one staff person to assist me, Gail Poe. I knew I would need to learn how to use the computer to manage the statistics, so I took a course offered by NCHS, led by Judy Fabrikant. At the conclusion of the course, the class celebrated, and, as often on other similar occasions, I wrote a piece for her.

Our Tribute to Judy Fabrikant

There was a young lady named Judy,
A model of feminine beauty.
But she's not only cute,
She can really compute
Well beyond the call of duty.

We all attended her class,
Hoping each of us would pass.
> *Now we manage our data*
> *From Alpha to Zeta*
Because we can call up SAS.

She taught us our JCL,
And our input and routing as well.
> *Nothing would faze her*
> *Not even the laser*
Or our questions, as dumb as Hell.
We learned about PROC PRINT and TABLES,
And run them as well as we're able
> *She showed us each error,*
> *Relieving our terror,*
And regaled us with computer fables.

We learned to insert and delete.
Running PROC FREQ was quite a feat.
> *The semicolon's a must,*
> *SAS will never adjust,*
Without it no line is complete.

They said the computer was dumb,
But I soon learned I was the one.
> *Judy taught us the rules,*
> *They're not friendly to fools.*
We persisted; we did not succumb.

Class is over. We reap what we sow.
We're amazed at what we know.

We will generate tables
With titles and labels
And Judy will bask in the glow.

I selected two broad areas for emphasis in the survey—behavior that reflected the role of prevention and care in the last year of life. NCHS had provided limited funds for the project, so I was required to raise a considerable sum from other federal agencies to fulfill our needs. I conferred with appropriate persons in most of the other units in the Public Health Service, including the National Cancer Institute, the National Heart and Lung Institute, the National Institute on Alcohol and Alcoholism, the National Institute of Mental Health, the National Institute on Aging, and the National Institute on Child Health and Human Development. I also approached the Social Security Administration, the Health Care Financing Agency, and the Veterans Administration. In all I secured about $2 million to supplement the NCHS funds. We contracted with the Bureau of the Census to conduct the mailings and interviews. We arranged for a second mailing if the first failed to produce a response, for telephone calls if both mailings failed, and for personal interviews as a last effort. We obtained an 86 percent response rate.

Managing the survey became complex. I was supervised by the chief of the Mortality Statistics Branch and got along well with him. He, in turn, was supervised by the director of the Division of Vital Statistics. The division director took little interest in the survey and seriously delayed responding to issues that needed his approval. I repeatedly complained but to no avail. In frustration I went to the new director of NCHS who succeeded Ms. Rice and described my concerns. I advised him that I would leave rather than continue under the impossible circumstance. I was in a position that I could, in fact, retire if needed. He recognized my concern and assigned a different supervisor who proved workable.

When the work of the survey was completed I wrote an article describing the major findings. The emphasis was on the high rate of disability among decedents in the last year of their life. *The Washington Post* published an article on page 1, and the Associated Press picked up the article. The NCHS clipping services sent me copies of about 100 articles in papers across the country crediting me for the findings.

With this assignment completed, I decided that it was time to retire.

THE PLAYWRIGHT
1970 (I WAS 54)

I never lost interest in the theatre. Shirley and I attended plays regularly. I kept the copy of my program for every play and made it a collection. Three full shelves on my bookcase held more than 1,000 programs of plays we attended. I decided to leave them to a theatre library as a collection. The Clarice Smith Performing Arts Center at the University of Maryland houses a Performing Arts Library, and they accepted the collection.

While still working at NCHS I decided it was time to try my hand at writing a play. I knew the theme I wanted to write on; it was about the first black mayor of a major American city. I took a week off, rented a cabin at Cacapon in West Virginia, took my Dictaphone machine, and spent a week in the cabin, dictating all day, taking my dinners at the restaurant at Cacapon. I returned home with several dictabelts and arranged to have them transcribed. When the work, *Dilemma*, was completed I sent off copies to several New York producers. I received a heartening response from one. He wrote that he would produce the play but for technical reasons having nothing to do with the play, he was not in a position to do so. I received no other responses.

After retiring I signed up to take a playwriting class with a playwright in the area who sponsored several courses. About six or eight of us came to class with scripts, portions were read, and we critiqued each other. I completed a second play, *Tomorrow and Tomorrow and Tomorrow*. It was the story of a television news anchor and his activist wife who worked at preventing nuclear war. The instructor arranged to have a reading with professional actors. The reading took place in a cold room in Alexandria, with few in attendance besides my family. It did not go over very well.

In part because I expected to do more playwriting and in part for vacation experiences, we bought a cabin in West Virginia at The Woods, between Martinsburg and Berkeley Springs.

THE CHANGING FAMILY
1960-1978

Our three "boys" grew older and went through their junior high and high school years. David took up the guitar and I drove him to his lessons. Jonny's interest in sports led him to the Boys Club. Jonny adopted the long hair that became more common, but his high school would not accept it. He transferred to Kennedy High School which was more liberal and more accepting. Philip took up drums, played in a neighborhood band and at school functions.

David was bar mitzvah at an orthodox congregation to please Shirley's father, who came to Washington for the occasion and stayed in a motel within walking distance of the "shul." Later we joined a conservative synagogue where Jonny was bar mitzvah. Philip studied for bar mitzvah with a private tutor and was bar mitzvah at the Cedar Lane Unitarian Church building.

What happened in the 1970s?
The Vietnam War ended.
The Soviet Union invaded Afghanistan.
President Nixon visited China.
The Metro began operation in the Washington area
The home computer was introduced
The Nuclear Non-proliferation Treaty went into effect.
The Beatles were in their prime.
The Pentagon Papers were released.

President Nixon resigned from the Presidency
after the Watergate scandal and cover-up.

David was eager to go to an Ivy League college. He chose Cornell, and Shirley and I visited each year for parents' weekends and other occasions. David began with an interest in mathematics but shifted to other interests. In his senior year he decided on psychology, and since he needed special courses, he stayed on for a fifth year. When he completed his degree, he married a classmate. He went to the University of Maryland for graduate work and obtained his Ph.D. He was divorced a few years later. His first employment was at the University of Iowa in Iowa City. While there he met a woman and married. The marriage lasted a few years and ended in divorce. A few years later he moved to a position on the counseling staff at Boston University. There he met Kathryn Jackson, a fellow psychologist, and they were married. Both worked at Boston University for some years; then Kathy took a position with Suffolk University, counseling and teaching. Both pursued creative and successful careers.

Jonny entered the University of Massachusetts in Boston. He had difficulty in adjustment there and returned home. Soon after, he got a bachelor's degree at the University of Maryland and then enrolled at American University for a graduate degree in public administration. He

Philip and his drums.

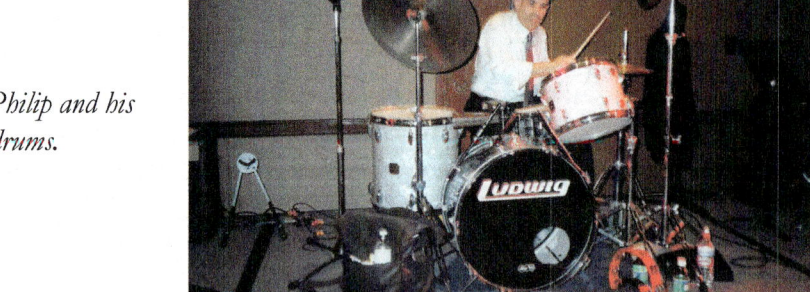

obtained employment at NIH for a time. Later he became active in politics, working for the election of Paris Glendening as county executive in Prince George's County. He joined the budget staff in Prince George's County. When Glendening was elected governor of Maryland, Jonny became

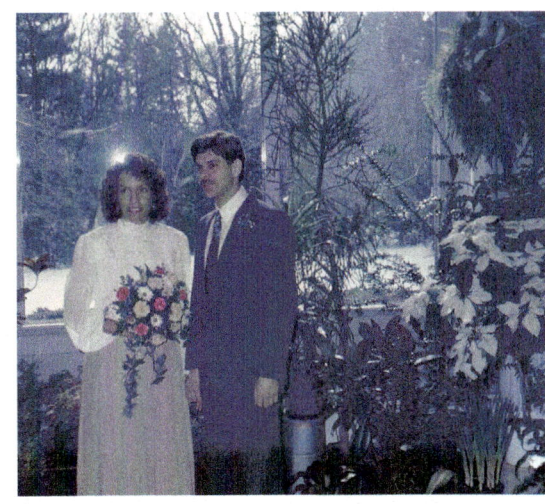

David and Kathy wed.

deputy secretary of the Maryland Department of Health and Mental Hygiene. Four years later a Republican was elected Maryland governor, and as a political appointee, Jonny was terminated. He then became head of the budget office in Prince George's County. This, too, was a political appointment, and after the next election, he was terminated. He took a budget position in Montgomery County but was not enthusiastic. He then became head of Finance and Budget for Queen Anne's County in Maryland.

Philip's interest in music led him to select Oberlin College in Ohio, where he continued his interest in drums and played in a band there. He majored in sociology and graduated. While there he developed a keen interest in computers and worked in the computer lab. When he graduated he was employed by the brother of a classmate who managed a hospital consultant business in Los Angeles, California. Soon he branched out, determined to work as an entrepreneur developing new software programs. He found creative ways to develop and market new programs. He also provided consultant services to managers and corporations.

My Brother Will's Death and Legacy
1982 (I was 66)

After Will's divorce, he continued to live and teach in Cincinnati, with his son Jeffrey living with him. In 1982 he was diagnosed with cancer of the pancreas, a disease with a very poor prognosis. Shirley and I visited him several times. At one point Will expressed an interest in visiting us in Silver Spring. I asked his physician if Will could make the plane trip, and his reply was, "Nothing could hurt him now".

We brought Will to our house for the visit, and we urged him to stay on. He agreed, and Shirley and I cared for him for weeks, until it became too difficult. We arranged for home hospice care. When even that was too much to manage, we arranged for him to be admitted to a hospice in Northern Virginia. He managed well there, with his apparent philosophical adjustment to his impending death. Shirley and I visited him every day at dinnertime. Will never spoke about his illness or coming death. I brought him a tape recorder and urged him to record his thoughts, hoping that he would complete the remainder of a psychobiography he had written years before. He never touched the recorder.

On September 11, 1982 Will died. Shirley and I were with him, and I held his hand when he drew his last breath. His son said that Will had expressed a desire to be cremated, and I arranged this. His ashes were to be buried in Cincinnati. Will meant so much to me that I arranged a memorial service for him at the University in Cincinnati. On my brother Mef's last visit to see Will, we sat around our kitchen table and Mef came up with the suggestion that the family establish a memorial fund in Will's name at the University. We readily agreed, and we established the William Seeman Psychology Research Fund. I carried his ashes on the plane to Cincinnati. At the funeral, I spoke about Will.

"I know that Will believed, as I believed most of my adult life, that we are mortal beings. Will has died, and all that remains of his mortal person we are now burying in the earth, to rest here eternally. Those of us who go on living will always know that Will rests here. But in these last weeks that I have been close to Will, as I knew he was dying, I had much time, and much need, to reflect on death and life, on mortality and immortality. My beliefs about immortality have changed.

That we are mortal is evident by what we are now doing—burying Will's mortal remains. That Will's immortality is evident and real and persistent and as stubborn as Will's spirit was in life is now clear to me, and I won't be argued out of it. Will's spark is in each of us who loved him and will go on loving him as long as each of us lives. That love does not end when we place these ashes in this earth.

But there is more to Will's immortality. Beyond each of us gathered here in whom Will's inspiration goes on living, there are all of those living students and teachers and scholars who were touched by Will's life. None of them is the same as they would have been had they not been burned by the flame of Will's life and work. Will's professorial passion has changed many people. Though he will no longer walk the streets of Cincinnati reading his books, his presence and his contribution will be felt in the halls and the classrooms at McMicken on campus.

To this evidence we also add the fruits of Will's scholarship which has been recorded and printed and will remain in university and clinical library shelves to be read and re-read through many years to come. Will's work is not mortal and is

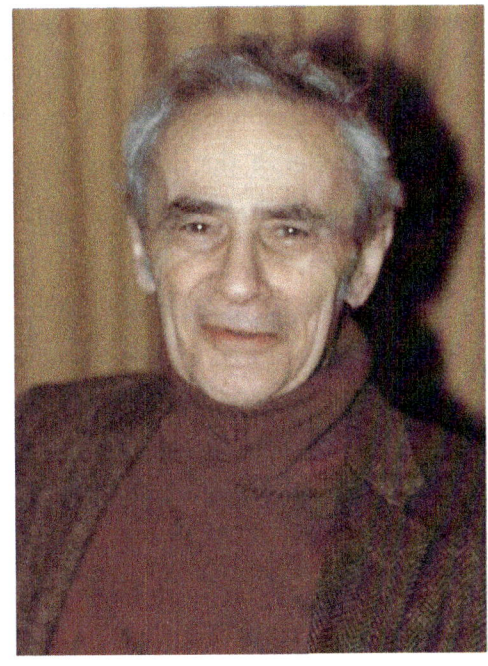

Will, who meant so much to me.

not buried here today. It will live.

And finally there is Will's living line of descent, Will's heritage to future generations, embodied in Jeffrey, Will's son. Much of Will lives on through Jeffrey.

For me, this reflection brings a small measure of comfort and peace, as I grieve for Will. I can believe and understand better that love I felt for Will all my life, and all of his life that I shared, the love that compelled Shirley and me to care for Will in our own way in these last months, is rewarded. Yes, there were difficult and rough and sad moments in these months but I can't describe the intensity of feeling for Shirley and for me that pervaded those hours at his bedside.

I can live now, with Will gone, not only because I must, since he was mortal, but with a new inspiration and a new passion for all the things Will stood for in my life, because they, too, will live on—the immortal Will.

I love what you lived for, Will, and I love you still—deeply."

You will know Will better from a fascinating incident that occurred three nights before he died. In the middle of the night Will rang the nurse's call bell at the hospice, and when the nurse, Cathy, came in, he said, "I have something urgent I want you to do. I have to write a check. In the top drawer of the cabinet you'll find a checkbook. Don't ask me to explain because it will take too long. I want you to write a check to Dr. Sigmund Freud."

When I spoke to Cathy later, she explained that, naturally enough, she was hesitant to follow his instruction, and she showed that reluctance. Will became impatient, even irritated. He said, "I know Sigmund Freud is dead. What I am not sure of is whether he died in 1940 or 1941. I want you to date that check before he died. Make it 1939. Make it out for $125, and I will sign it."

I retain one of my most precious possessions, a check that associates my brother William Seeman with Dr. Sigmund Freud. I prepared a pamphlet in Will's honor.

A Larger Family

Philip met Diane Levy and they were married in Rochester, N.Y. but Philip with his new bride continued to live in California. Diane was trained as a physical therapist, working with very young children. Shirley and I visited often, especially when their daughter Laura was born and later when Anna was born.

> *In January 1989, George H. W. Bush was inaugurated as president of the United States.*

Shirley and I were introduced to this new experience as grandparents.

Soon after Laura was born, I wrote an:

ODE TO LAURA

A child of my child and his recent bride is newborn.
She is a miracle of the miracle of life.
Nurtured in mother's womb, under father's watchful eye,
> *From a woman's seed, in union with the seed of man,*
> *And born in the eternal chain of generation after genera-*
tion after generation of peoplehood.
An heir of all mankind that has gone before, and destined to bear
a generation beyond.

Yet she is Laura--unique, unmatched, new, and different,
Different from all who have lived and died.
She is Laura--special, and all her own,
> *Her own special eyes searching her tiny world,*
> *Her own lovely face, flailing arms, legs exploring the air.*
Her own charm, her own grace, her own joy of life.

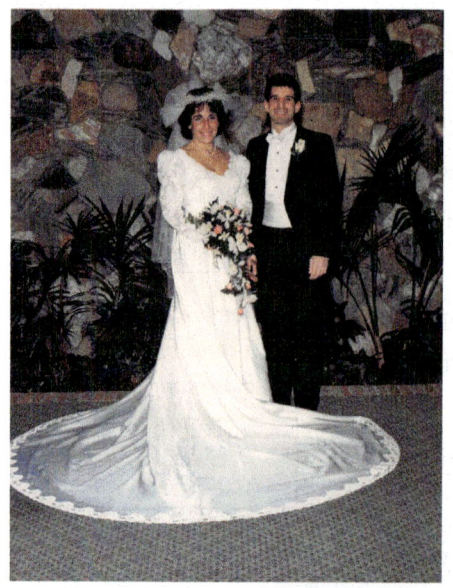

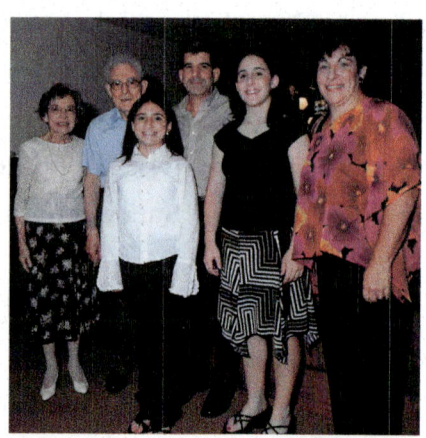

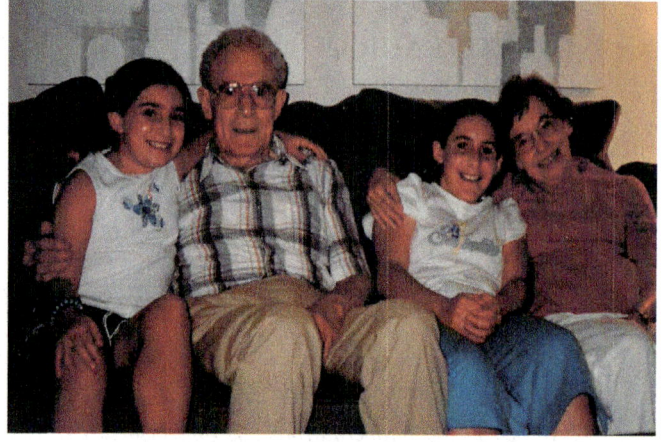

Clockwise from above:

Philip and Diane wed.

A larger family.

Grandparents and grandchildren.

Laura and Annie.

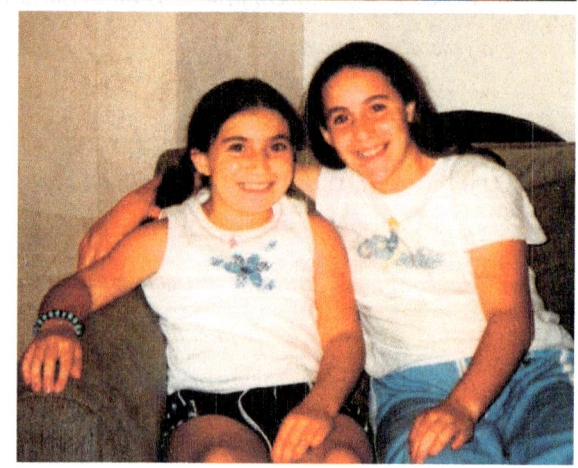

Laura fills a unique place in the history of this world,
For I am the child of my father and mother, who each had a mother
and father,
　　　　And I had a child who is now father to my grandchild,
And she is Laura.

My child bears my seed   into the next generation,
And his seed spawns the generations beyond,
And the generations shall go on.
Thus I come from the past, yet I shall go on – through Laura.

Laura is the miracle of life.
Laura is the joy of living.
Laura is at peace, the peace of innocence.
Laura is the hope of life and joy and peace.

When Annie was born, somehow I delayed my celebration until she was about two years old. Then I wrote –

ANNIE AND HER BOOKS

Annie is an open book.
What you see is what she is.
Pure, genuine, honest joy.

Annie is an open book.
And her book is always open.
Annie loves books, and books love Annie.
Offer to read to her – a book,
Or don't offer, and she will bring the book to you.

Not one book, but books.
Books she loves.

When all else fails, there is a book for Annie.
There are favorites, and there are those that pass quickly.
But make it a book.

Bring her a book, and Annie will smile.
That broad, beautiful, warm, loving smile.
It is contagious, Annie's smile.
Read to her, and the smile goes on.

She drinks in the words, and gives them back to you.
She swallows the pictures, and shows them back to you.

You do not need to read to Annie,
She will read to herself.
All of age two, and she reads her books to herself — or to you.
But to herself is best.

Annie is a joy.
Annie is a smile.
Annie is entirely herself.
Annie and her books.
Annie is an open book.
Read and enjoy her.

Jonny married a long-time friend, but the marriage did not last and they were divorced. When Jonny was working in Maryland he met Laura Healy, an employee in the Maryland State Department of Occupational Safety and Health, and they were married. Laura had a daughter, Sarah, and Jonny quickly developed a good relationship with her. A few years later they had a son, James, our third grandchild.

Ode to James Michael Seeman

Our heritage will go on.
Today my son had a son, my grandson, James Michael Seeman.
The son of Jonathan Seeman and Laura Healy Seeman.
And Jonathan is my son.
The line will go on--the Seeman line.

I am the son of my father, who had a father.
I am the father of my son, who is now a father.
Today, the heritage of the long past is the heritage of the future.

My grandson will grow, a child in the Seeman line.
His father will teach him the ways of the world, and his mother will nurture him to manhood.
He will become a father to his sons, in the Seeman line.

Today is a joyous day.
There is another Seeman in the family of Seemans--James Michael.
Today is a day of rejoicing and celebration.

Jonny and Laura wed.

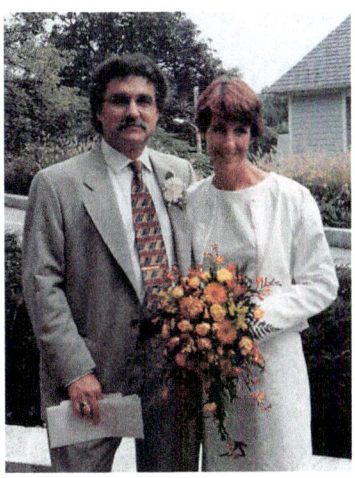

Laura later transferred to the U.S. Department of Labor, still in Occupational Safety and Health. After some years, she was promoted to a senior position. Later, the two divorced.

What happened in the 1980s?
The nuclear accident in Chernobyl occurred.
The oil spill from the Exxon Valdez took place.
Anwar Sadat of Egypt was assassinated.
The Berlin Wall fell.
There was a massacre at Tiananmen Square in China.
The attempt to rescue the hostages in Iran failed.
The first woman was appointed to the Supreme
Court —Sandra Day O'Connor.
The AIDS epidemic began.
The Iran-Contra scandal took place.

THE RECONSTRUCTIONIST HAVURAH OF GREATER WASHINGTON AND ADAT SHALOM RECONSTRUCTIONIST CONGREGATION
1991

Our friends the Goldblatts (I had recruited Harold from New York to serve with HWC) repeatedly invited us to meetings of a study and discussion group that they enjoyed, the Reconstructionist Havurah of Greater Washington. After some time, Shirley and I attended several meetings, and we joined. We met each month and discussed books or topics related to

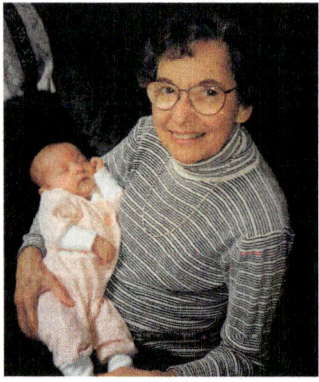
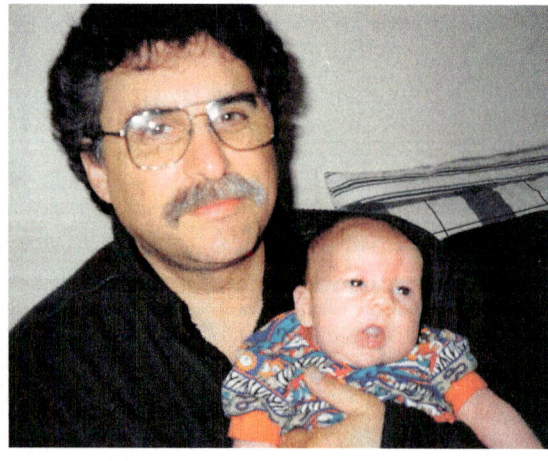

Above: Shirley and Jamie.
Right: Jonny and Jamie.

Reconstructionism or Judaism. After a few years I was elected president. With almost all of the other members having served as president there were few who agreed to serve. I continued as president for more than 15 years.

Shirley and I had not been members of a congregation since Jonny's bar mitzvah. We did not find one we felt comfortable with. Shirley particularly had a problem based on her experience with her extremely religious father. One day she saw a notice of a group that planned to hold a Reconstructionist High Holiday service. We attended and found the Rabbi, Sid Schwartz, and the service worthwhile. The group then led to the formation of a new congregation, Adat Shalom Reconstructionist Congregation. We joined and attended services periodically. I continue my membership but attend seldom. The services are interactive and interesting, but involve a great deal of "davening" (repeating the prayers) which does not appeal to me.

What happened in the 1990s?

Iraq invaded Kuwait, and the Desert Storm war forced a withdrawal.
Nelson Mandela was freed from prison after 27 years.
The first World Trade Center bombing occurred.
The World Wide Web was inaugurated.
Carol Mosley Braun was the first black woman elected to the Senate.
The Oklahoma City Federal Building was bombed.
The Palestinians were given limited self-rule in a White House signing.
Princess Diana was killed in an auto accident.
The first cloning of a sheep, Dolly, occurred.
A peace agreement was signed in Northern Ireland.

The Metropolitan Washington
Public Health Association
1999-2001

After retiring, I attended a meeting of the Metropolitan Washington Public Health Association. This organization evolved from the D.C. association of which I was a charter member. At the meeting I sat next to a woman who was very active and who was on the nominating committee. When I told her I had just retired, she said they needed me to become president of the association. After some thought, I agreed. I served as president for a one-year term.

At the end of my term, the president-elect who would succeed me moved out of the area, so I served a second year as president. I made some changes in the structure and achieved several other initiatives. I recruited a student at the School of Public Health and Health Services at George Washington University, and with his help we undertook a statistical project. Using a set of public health objectives published by the U.S. Department of Health and Human Services, I gathered data for each of the six jurisdictions in the area on each of 26 objectives and published the results as the public health indicators. I also arranged a conference to release the results. I continued to work with MWPHA for many years after.

> *In January 1993, Bill Clinton was inaugurated as president of the United States.*

What happened in the 2000s?

The attack on the World Trade Center and the Pentagon took place on September 11, 2001.
The U.S. invaded Afghanistan and Iraq.
The U.S. Supreme Court decided the election of George W. Bush.
The Euro currency was introduced.
Hurricane Katrina devastated New Orleans.

Barack Obama was the first African American elected President.
The Human Genome project was completed.
The Enron Corporation went into bankruptcy.

RSVP Times Two
1985 (I was 69)

While I was retired, Shirley found a new vocation. She was employed by Montgomery County as a counselor with the Retired Senior Volunteer Program (RSVP). She matched seniors interested in volunteer work with agencies that needed volunteers. While there were administrative hitches in the agency, she found the work very worthwhile and rewarding. She developed good relationships with several of the other staff members.

During this period Shirley turned 75. I decided I would arrange a surprise birthday party for her. I prepared a list of invitees and wrote invitations in calligraphy, with an RSVP, but informed the invitees that it was a surprise, and gifts were not required. I ordered the food. David came down from Cambridge, and he and I took Shirley to an art museum, so Jonny could come to the house and lay out the food. We drove Shirley back in time for the party. As we approached the house she noticed many cars, and commented that our next door neighbors, the Fishmans, must be having a party. She entered the house and was truly surprised.

A Working Retirement
1986 (I was 70)

I kept in touch with the NCHS office after retiring. A 1993 Mortality Followback Survey was being planned, and I served as a consultant. I received a contract to test parts of the new survey, especially with regard to homicide and suicide. I interviewed a small sample of the next of kin of persons who had died of these causes to test the questionnaire.

The Metropolitan Washington Public Health
ASSESSMENT CENTER
1999-2001 (I WAS 83-85)

After completing the work on the public health indicators, I saw the need to continue this effort. With funding from NCHS arranged by an associate I had worked with, and with support from the Dean of the School at George Washington University, I established the Metropolitan Washington Public Health Assessment Center. I secured the cooperation of the Health Officials Committee of the Metropolitan Washington Council of Governments. I established a Policy and Management Committee of which I was elected chairman.

Staffing of the center was provided by the chairman of the school's Department of Epidemiology and Biostatistics, an aide, and two students. With the cooperation of the nine health jurisdictions included in COG, we prepared an updated and thoroughly professional report on health indictors for the metropolitan region. Publication of the report was funded by the Group Health Foundation and the Northern Virginia Health Foundation. This report was presented at a special meeting, at which the president of Kaiser Permanente for the Mid-Atlantic States and the chairman of the COG committee honored me with a life-time achievement award.

I had hoped to continue the center, but when the chair of the Epidemiology and Biostatistics Department left the school, and funds were depleted, the center became dormant.

With support from a small sum still available from NCHS for a contract, I continued the effort to keep the center functioning, I served as a central point for gathering data from each of the jurisdictions on the incidence of West Nile Virus infection, a new outbreak in the area, and the collection of dead birds and the trapping of mosquitoes. I also found other interests relevant to the center's functions. The new chair of the

Department of Epidemiology and Biostatistics, while expressing interest in the center, took no action unless I could find funding. The center failed to continue.

THE KAISER PERMANENTE EXPERIENCE
1995

When we moved to the Washington area we needed to select a health plan. Without hesitation I chose Group Health, a co-op plan. It worked out well for us for many years, but in time we found the administrative aspects unsatisfactory, e.g., getting through on the phone and getting appointments. I switched plans and enrolled in the Georgetown University Health Plan. Soon after we enrolled, the Georgetown plan was purchased by Kaiser Permanente, and we were now members of Kaiser. We found this plan worked well for us.

One day I saw a notice in a bulletin from Kaiser that they had a Member Advisory Council, and our Kensington Center was holding an election for two members. I submitted my nomination, and I was elected. In addition to meeting at the center, I also served on the Regional Council. I became quite active, and when a regional election for chairman was occurring, the staff person urged me to run. I did so and was elected chairperson of the Regional Council. This proved to be a most interesting but difficult assignment. There were two members who dominated discussions and always about their personal health which was not the purpose of the Advisory Council. I struggled through it and was elected for a second term as chairperson.

The Kaiser bylaws provided that two members of the Advisory Council were elected to serve on the Mid-Atlantic Board of Directors. I was nominated for one of these positions and was elected. I was now serving on the Kaiser Board, a very challenging and rewarding opportunity. I was very active during a period when the board faced serious issues. I

128

served on the board for eight years. I continued to serve on the Member Advisory Council, until the Kaiser president, Marilyn Kawamura, found the council to be unproductive and over several years she reduced its role and ultimately abandoned the council. I continued to maintain contact with the president and several other key staff.

During this time I became acquainted with a member of the Permanente Board (the medical group) who was director of research for Permanente. He invited me to become a member of the Mid-Atlantic Institutional Review Board and I agreed. I served in this capacity for about 10 years and found it educational and interesting. I served as a community member which IRB's are required to have at each meeting. During this time I was informed that Holy Cross Hospital was seeking a community member for their IRB, and invited me to join. I did so and served on both IRBs until retiring from both at about age 95.

Throughout my life I held the view that each of us gets two lives to live—one the professional and one the personal. For the professional, to succeed we must have insight, training, skill, judgment, and perseverance. For the personal, we must have patience, understanding, compassion, forgiveness, and sacrifice.

At the Heights, To My Love

I know, at last, I now have reached the height
Of all I ever hoped and dreamed I might.

I pause, as pause I must before I die,
To take account of who I am, this I.

This one, this only I ever drew breath,
This I, at reckoning before inevitable death.

Where have I been, what have I done on earth,
Through countless hours and days, years since my birth?

The time has come to assess the good, the bad,
To learn if I must sing for joy, or go so sad.

I take the measure of the years I've spent,
To learn if I rejoice, or must repent.

In this last judgment I must know the truth.
No hasty summing, no rash guess of youth.

The answer comes to me, quite loud and clear.
Where I do stand, I stand without doubt or fear.

One credo throughout this life was ever my
guide,
An ethic I'd proclaim, not hide.

In January 2001,
George W. Bush
was inaugurated as
president of the
United States.

When you do leave this earth to which you
came,
You must not go and leave it just the same.

Leave it a better place because you were here.
What is your legacy, solemn, sincere?

This world is far too wide, too vast
To change, to turn quite different from the past.

Therefore , fix firmly in your sights,
The vision you would see from new-won heights,

Bring change to only one, one whom you love,
Look down on only one from skies above.

If, when the game is done, you truly know,
Your mission complete, as from this earth you go.

She whom you loved, once troubled, once quite sad
From childhood, more tears than joy has had,

She whose life you life-long deeply shared,
She, whose outlook on this life you dared

To change, to move from pain to joy,
Through deepest love you did employ,

To wipe away the tears, the fears, the negative,
Replaced by happy days, accepting the love you give.

New brighter joys, new loving ways,
Two happy souls living out their well-earned days

In understanding, sharing, passionate twin embrace,
Drinking in the pleasures of this pleasant place.

Look back upon both joy and anguish known,
And see fruits of the seed you've sown.

One person on this earth you gave all love.
She, from her depths, did truly rise above.

She and you, once two, through love became but one.
Then know, this earthly game you've won.

SHIRLEY'S ILLNESS AND DEATH
2004-2005 (I WAS 88 TO 89)

In 2004 Shirley noticed a swelling in the area of her neck. She made an appointment with an otolaryngologist, Dr. Sclarew. He was uncertain what the problem was, and advised her to have a biopsy of the swelling. They took a fine-needle biopsy which proved inconclusive. They repeated the biopsy and made a diagnosis of non-Hodgkin's lymphoma. She made an appointment with an oncologist. He recommended the standard treatment for indolent non-Hodgkin's lymphoma, a watch and wait plan. At this time no active therapy was recommended. She asked him how long she might have to live with this condition. He asked how long she wanted, and when she said ten years, he said, "You've got it." That proved not to be accurate.

Shirley felt uncomfortable with this oncologist. He was very low-key and not very communicative. She made an appointment with another oncologist, Dr. Leon Hwang, whom I knew because he served on the IRB. He sought further information and referred her to an oncologist at Johns Hopkins Hospital who was the investigator on a clinical trial. He examined Shirley and found a lump in the groin area. She had a biopsy which led to a change in the diagnosis. It was concluded that she had Hodgkin's lymphoma. Dr. Hwang wished to undertake chemotherapy but felt Shirley needed to gain strength first. He recommended a regimen to strengthen her. After a period, he concluded that she would be unable to receive therapy. I vividly recall that conference with him. He informed her that there was nothing that could be done. When Shirley asked, he said she had six months to live. When he left, Shirley and I stood, hugged each other, and cried.

Before this diagnosis we had decided that it was time to sell the house on Dameron Drive where we had lived for over 50 years, and move to a retirement community. We explored several and decided to move to Riderwood Village in Silver Spring. We moved in August 2005.

Shirley's health deteriorated. We enrolled in the Montgomery Hospice to aid in her care, and they proved very helpful. In time I employed an agency to provide aid to Shirley. She was naturally depressed. Several times she said she was not a good mother. I challenged this observation. I arranged for each of our sons to visit her and tell her what a good mother she was.

One night she awoke and said, "I love you so much." I shall never forget that moment.

In January 2006 the Hospice nurse informed us that death was near. I arranged for David to come to Silver Spring from Cambridge. On the morning of January 23 I called Jonny and Philip to come to the apartment. It was clear she was near death, but we believe she waited until Jonny came. She died that morning. I cried.

REMEMBERING SHIRLEY

A quiet, lonely, and sad period followed. That first night or two I stayed at Philip's house; I could not be alone. Returning to an empty apartment was difficult. The loneliness hung over the days and nights. Going to the dining room alone was unpleasant. I wrote poems, several poems, and articles to relieve the depression. Each time I spoke with someone about her I cried. The Hospice provided a bereavement nurse with whom I became very friendly, and she was most helpful. She appreciated one of the articles I wrote about my loneliness and had it published in the Hospice newsletter.

I had a tree planted at Riderwood in Shirley's memory, close to the garage where I could see it every time I used the car or walked nearby.

Unfortunately, it died because it was a dogwood in too much sun. I had another dogwood planted nearby.

I put Shirley's wedding ring and my wedding ring on my keychain so I could feel them every time I locked or unlocked the apartment door. When Adat Shalom, my congregation, opened a walkway with memorial stones engraved as memorials, I had one placed for Shirley.

Flowers on Her Grave

I placed flowers on her grave today.
I know she does not know.
But I know.

Half a year ago we lowered her into her grave;
We covered the coffin with earth,
The earth I now touch to be as near to her as I can be.

My thoughts are wholly with her,
My voice speaks to her because I know.
I know I must tell her how much I love her still,
She must know how I miss her each day.

I was drawn to her grave today.
I placed flowers on her grave,
And spoke to her, in my way.
I know.

CELEBRATING MY 90TH
(2006)

Diane and Philip arranged a 90th birthday party at their house in North Potomac. We invited family and friends, and people I had worked with over the years. I spoke about each one, commenting on what my relationship had been with each. It was a heartwarming affair.

What is happening in the 2010s?
Haiti was hit by a severe earthquake.
There were riots in Greece.
North Korea announced it had nuclear weapons.
The U.S. and Russia reached an agreement to limit nuclear arms.
The B.P. oil spill occurred.

THE INSTITUTE FOR SCIENCE AND JUDAISM

I developed a friendly relationship with Rabbi George Driesen, auxiliary Rabbi at Adat Shalom, and he led the funeral service for Shirley. One Rosh Hashanah he presented a sermon on the relationship of science and Judaism. Soon after, he organized an agency to present discussions on this topic. He invited me to join the Board of Directors.

Since I am away from Maryland six months of the year, I am not very active with the organization. It has presented some very interesting speakers on the subject.

Looking Back

Now I cannot tell her how deeply I loved her--and love her still.
Her body lies beneath this small plot of earth where I stand.
She cannot see my tears, hear my weeping, feel my grief.

Did I tell her, when I could, of my love?
Why did I not, when I should, grasp her close to my breast?
Did I ask her to forgive my anger and my harsh words?
Did I say am I sorry when I should?

I look back with painful regrets,
But I cannot go back.
Go back and say what should have been said,
Do what should have been done.

Hurt as it will, the past is passed, and cannot be relived.
She cannot know how deeply I regret.
I whispered of my love that should have been shouted.

Now I stand here and tell the heavens and the earth
What I cannot tell her.

SHIRLEY'S SISTER, ADA RHEA
1949-2011

Ada Rhea, Shirley's sister, had a very troubled life. Her eldest son, Rickey, was killed in a plane crash on his way back to college. Her daughter, Julie, was born with a mental disability, experienced innumerable diagnostic encounters, required special education and ultimately lives in a farm community in Virginia. Ada Rhea's husband, Ernest, later filed for divorce after meeting another woman.

Shirley and I drove her to Wilmington, DE where her divorce lawyer resided. Not long after, her ex-husband died. After the divorce she returned to work, employed by the World Bank. During all the years that she was alone, we saw her often. I took over the management of her finances and investments and continued this for years. Shirley met her often, trying to ease her life and also trying to improve her outlook which was serious depression. After Shirley died, I arranged for Ada Rhea to move from a dingy basement apartment to a senior retirement home run by the Jewish Federation.

Ada Rhea fell one day and was taken to the emergency department at Suburban Hospital. There an x-ray was taken and revealed advanced lung cancer, which had spread to other organs. We had no knowledge of this and there were no symptoms. She left the hospital and entered the Hebrew Home. I visited her there regularly. I had many contacts with her son, Andy, who lived in New York. She lived for about six months and died in 2011.

I EMBRACE BEETHOVEN
2004 (I WAS 88)

I had always had a passion for the music of Beethoven. Around this time I picked up a copy of a biography of Beethoven by Maynard Solomon and read it. I took notes as I read and found his great music matched by a fascinating and difficult life. I read several other biographies.

I decided to write a one-man play on his life and work, and I did so. When it was edited and complete, I approached the television studio at Riderwood and asked if they would film me playing the part of Beethoven. I gave them the script, and they agreed. I studied the part over a lengthy period. I called a friend who had been artistic director of Round House Theatre hoping he would direct me in the play, but having gone independent, he needed to add to his income, so it did not work out.

The play was written in four acts. We filmed part I, I studied part II, and we filmed it, and on to parts III and IV. I arranged for an evening in the chapel to advertise the upcoming production, and arranged for a violinist and pianist to play a Beethoven sonata. It was well attended. Soon after, each act was broadcast on Riderwood TV a week apart. I also had several DVDs made, and showed the play to friends. I gave copies to several music instructors who made favorable comments.

MARILYN REAPPEARS
2005 (I WAS 89)

And we join hearts.

Before Shirley died I was working on the computer one day when a pop-up appeared. I always ignored pop-ups, but somehow this one attracted my attention. It described an opportunity for a cruise to the Bahamas with reduced rates at hotels en route. I thought it would be good to take Shirley on the cruise, so I responded. With a payment I received a coupon for the trip. Shirley never felt up to the trip. I learned that I could hold the coupon for two years.

Shirley and I had attended two Elderhostel sessions at Peabody Conservatory in Baltimore. Now alone, I saw a notice of a new session there with all three classes on Beethoven. I decided to make the trip.

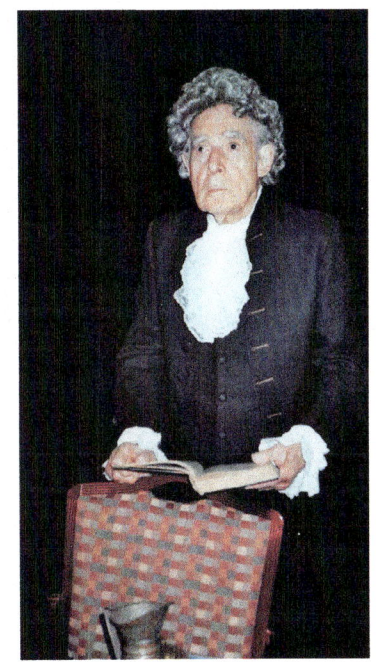

While there I asked the Elderhostel host if I could read my Beethoven play one evening, and he agreed. The performance was advertised with notices around the building.

After the performance, Marilyn Willner, whom I had met years before when she lived across the street and

I become Beethoven.

became well acquainted with Shirley wheeling their babies together, came up and reintroduced herself. She had seen the notice of the performance and recognized the name Isadore Seeman.

She inquired at the desk whether I was accompanied by my wife, and was informed that I was not. Her husband, Dr. David Willner, had died.

When she reintroduced herself, I learned that she was living in Florida. I asked for her address and phone number, which she gave me.

Months went by. One day, still alone, I decided it was time to take the cruise to the Bahamas. The arrangement included a stay at a hotel in Orlando, and the ship left from Ft. Lauderdale. I realized I would be passing Delray Beach where Marilyn lived. I called to ask if we could have lunch together on my route. She agreed. A few days later I called again and told her I could get separate hotel rooms, and asked if she would like to accompany me on the cruise. Again she agreed.

I stopped in Delray Beach, had lunch with Marilyn, and we set out for the rest of the trip. As it turned out, the low price for the trip was based on the requirement for me to listen three times to a sales pitch to buy time shares. I listened but made no purchase.

Marilyn and I enjoyed the trip. The night before we were to part I told her that I forgot to tell her that I loved her. We agreed to meet again.

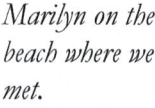

Marilyn on the beach where we met.

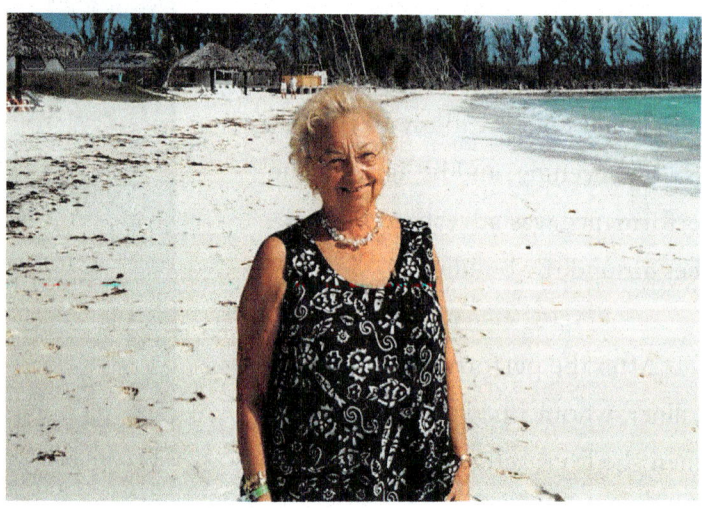

We discussed living arrangements. We agreed that marriage was not a part of the arrangement. We also agreed that our assets would not be mingled. She owned a condo in Delray Beach, Florida and a condo in Ventnor, N.J. I owned the unit at Riderwood. We agreed to spend winters in Florida, spring and fall in Silver Spring, and summers in Ventnor.

I was accepted by her family: There was her sister, Sheila, and her brother-in-law, Albie. In fact Albie and I developed a close, warm relationship. There was her daughter Rachel, and son-in-law Ron, and the grandchildren, Danny and Ariel. We visited them and enjoyed new family. And there is her son, Shep, who has accepted me generously. She was well received by my family.

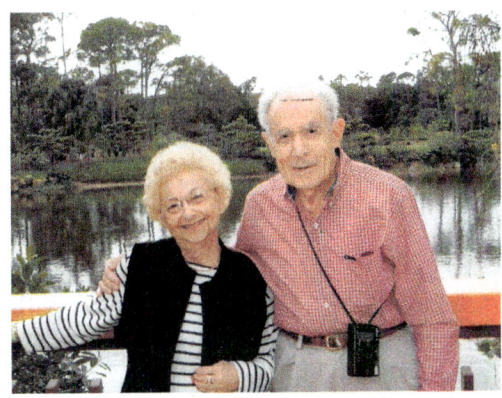

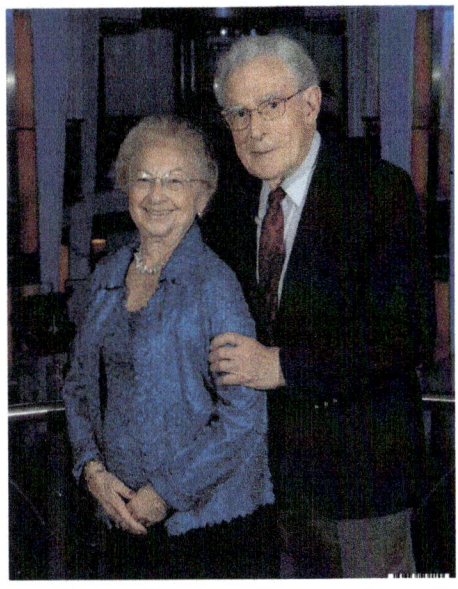

Top: Marilyn and me.
Above: Marilyn and me on a cruise.

We Two

Two paths are open to each of us.
We can choose, as most do, to find a mate — one who enriches our lives, with whom we spend our years together, with its joys and its trials, yet in all, a wondrous journey.
Or we can live alone, in all, a lonely journey.

All too often, on this path, as years go by, that awesome phrase each has spoken to the other in our union—"'till death do us part"—becomes real, and once again, one is alone. Most often it is she, alone. Visit any of the many communities of retirement, and observe those alone--she most often.

> *In January 2009, Barack Obama was inaugurated as the first African American president of the United States.*

Two paths are again open to each of us, though less open than the paths of youth.

How fortunate, then, are we, to have found each other, Marilyn and Sam. Those lonely years, those times of solitude, are behind us. We are now two who have found each other.

Learning, again, how to live together. Is she without flaw? Am I? All that we have learned and lived over the long years is still with each of us. So we learn again, of life for two—sharing, caring, forgiving, and yes, new love.

To Marilyn

When she and he together share this life,
Knowing they must endure what fate decrees,
Prepared to suffer pain, tragedy, and strife,
To weather cold and dark stormy seas.

Yet filled with hope instead, great joy to know,
From stress and trial and pressure find surcease,
To plant the seeds of happiness, to grow,
From all that may befall to find calm peace.

Then know the immutable law decreed above,

Life is a journey meant for two,
At heart all that befalls depends on love,
And love knows but one master--you.

If you'd be loved, that love yourself must earn,
Only the love you give comes back in rich return.

IN MEMORY OF JULES
2011

Jules died in 2011. I recall the bitter cold day when we buried him. Not long after, his devoted wife Mar (Marilyn) organized a memorial service. I spoke there.

"Jules was many things to very many people. I treasure a unique relationship—I was his brother. Brothers are special, and Jules was special. Jules was a good brother.

Brothers talk to each other in ways different than with all others. They experience common life events. They see things differently than friends and colleagues and others. And Jules was a good brother.

Most of you probably think Jules was a serious guy. But that's because you never played mumbley-peg with Jules. You never played caddie with Jules, or home sheep run, or shot hoodles. I did. You never went with him on Saturday to a 5-cent movie, to see Hoot Gibson or Tom Mix, the western cowboys. I did. And Jules was a lot of fun.

Our family was Mom and Pop and four brothers and one sister. We four brothers were a close clan. We were well known around Baltimore—the Seeman boys. Often if one of us went to the Ford's Theatre in Baltimore and sat up in the cheapest seats in the second balcony, all four of us were there. There were years when all four of the Seeman brothers were elementary school teachers in the Baltimore City public schools. It's pretty hard to match that.

We were children of the depression. Our father was a shoemaker, never very successful in business. We moved 10 times in Baltimore. When Pop's shoe repair didn't bring in a living, he tried a grocery store, a liquor store, a restaurant, a second hand clothing store, and we always lived upstairs, once without an inside toilet.

Our father had little use for education. It made more sense for the boys to go to work and bring in some money for the family. And work we did, every one of the boys while we were in high school. Jules spotted a street corner in downtown Baltimore and made that his news-stand. He sold the *Baltimore Sun*, the *News*, and the *Post*. He hopped the street cars to sell paper to the riders. I have a vivid memory of one bitter cold winter night when Jules came home after a day on the corner, his feet almost frozen. Our mother heated water and poured it into a basin for Jules to soak his feet and warm up.

Our mother had a very different view of education. To her it was life's goal. She was determined to see her children educated, in spite of our poverty and our father's opposition. So instead of a four-year college, our oldest brother Will went to State Normal School, and worked under Roosevelt's National Youth Administration to earn the fifty dollar tuition, and in two years he was a teacher. Jules followed with a three-year diploma, and then Mef and me. But then Will studied further, and was very proud when he got his Ph.D. In fact, our mother produced three Ph.Ds, and three university professors, Jules among them.

Jules

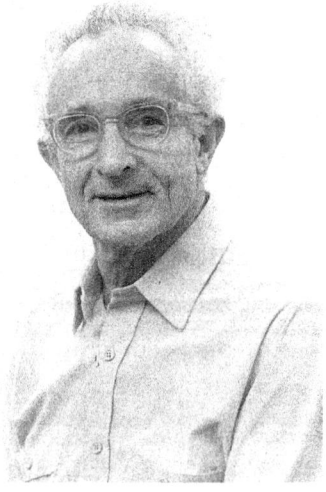

But Jules was Jules. He was not Will, and not Mef. He was Jules. Jules was always organized. When the brothers began working after school and week-ends and bringing money into the house, it was Jules who kept the family books—income and outlay. We were a socialist family—from each according to his ability and to each according to his need. And Jules kept the financial record.

The brothers sometimes went out on double dates, and Jules introduced us to a sedate young woman, Esther Millon. Very bright, very intellectual. Jules married Esther, and chief among the results were Larry and Brad. I remember a visit to Jules and Esther in Chicago, where we heard their philosophy of child-rearing. It was child-centered and permissive, so much so that they allowed Larry to eat only the one food he liked. We were a bit shocked at that.

Later Jules and Esther came home from their many trips abroad, regaling us with the great adventures they had had. Esther introduced us to a foreign country named Japan, when she was Executive Director of the Japan Center of Tennessee.

Jules was just 16 months older than I. After more than 90 birthdays, I was never able to catch up to him. That applies in many ways. I could never catch up to his original and creative ways to interpret psychology. I was never able to catch up to his articles and his books and his awards. Although I was a brother to Jules, there were times when I felt I was a patient. He reinterpreted what we were discussing in a manner only Jules could do. After reading *The Case of Jim*, I began to think I was the case of Isadore.

Jules was a good brother. Throughout our working years, he often passed investment advice to me. Most often it was good advice, and I profited from it, but it could occasionally be bad advice, too. There was a time when, on Jules' advice, all of the Seeman brothers bought condo units in Panama City Beach in Florida for investment. Before too long, all of us went into foreclosure.

I am now at a time in my life when I think of legacy. Jules leaves a very very rich legacy—his students, his colleagues, his patients, his associations, his articles and books, and most important his family—his wife Mar, his sons Larry and Brad, his grandchildren and great grandchildren.

I loved my brothers and my sister. I spoke of my love for Will at his memorial service. I spoke of my love for Gussie at her memorial service. I am here to attest, to attest that I loved Jules.

Jules owes me a debt he never paid. The close family knows the story well. When we were children, the four brothers paired off in different ways. At times, I was closest to Will, at times to Jules. Will and Jules as the two oldest were often closest. One day the two of them wanted to go off and do things little brothers can't do. So they sat Mef and me down on the steps in front of 1922 Fleet Street in Baltimore. To keep us from tagging along, they promised us that when they returned they would bring us a pony. Will died some years ago, but during his lifetime he never showed the slightest sign of bringing that pony. Now, today, I know that Mef and I will never get that pony."

Life Takes Its Toll

When my brother Mef met Alice Zerbola at Teachers College and they started dating, he knew that he needed some way to keep our parents from knowing he was dated a non-Jew. He began calling her Jake. That name lasted through the years.

They were a beautiful couple, living in a lovely house overlooking the Pacific. Late in life, Alice had a stroke, a very difficult experience, but she was serious about managing and rehab. Some years later Alice died, and Mef was devastated as we shared a common experience.

I Reach 99
(2014)

I have set down in words an account of my life. It covers 99 years. The latest data on the expectation of life for an American male is 75 years; when I was born it was 50 years for a white male. I have outlived the average. As each birthday passes we add only one year; accumulating years to 99 brings a sense of wonder—how did I get to 99? Does it feel like 99?

People ask me: to what do you attribute your longevity. I honestly don't know. I know that genes play a major role. My father lived to his 80s; my mother died in her 70s but an automobile intervened, so we don't know how long she might have lived. Will died at 70; Jules at 95. Diet and exercise surely play a part, and I have been reasonably attentive and active. More I cannot say.

> In January 2013, Barack Obama was sworn in for a second term as president of the United States.

A more important question is, not how long I lived, but how well. On this point I have a response. Each of us, to live well, must discover or develop a passion, and relentlessly pursue that passion. This can bring fulfillment. My passion? Several. To serve the community. To help make my family happy. The theatre. And to relate sincerely and well to friends and all others. These are my passions.

I reflect on all that I have lived through, what I have done, what left undone; what worked and what failed; what I accomplished and what I should have done dif- *Alice and Mef* ferently. I seek a perspective, an assessment. It is time to consider the legacy.

In my professional career—

• I am most proud of my work at HWC as an agent of community change and social advancement. I was a community leader. I contributed modestly to civil rights. I recruited African Americans for leadership roles in HWC and developed close relation-

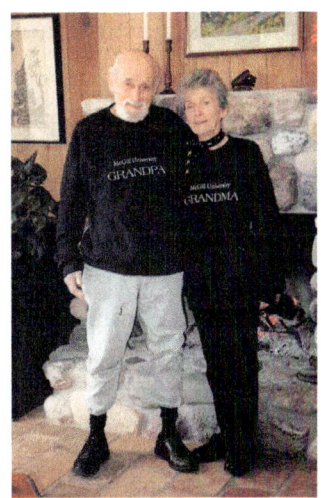

ships with them. I created the Metropolitan Washington Child Day Care Association, the Metropolitan Washington Homemaker Service; the Health and Welfare Council of the National Capital Area; the United Planning Organization; although transient, the Metropolitan Washington Public Health Assessment Center. Most of these programs continue to meet needs today. The Community Health Indicators study I initiated continues regularly.

- I successfully managed the 1986 National Mortality Followback Survey. It revealed data that proved informative for the public and a useful resource for further study and research.

- As executive director of the Health and Welfare Council for 18 years, I supervised the allocation of about $180 million to community service agencies and managed the organization with responsibility and accountability.

- I thoroughly enjoyed my work in the theatre. The several plays I wrote did not measure up to production level, but I relished the effort. I did produce and act in the Beethoven play. I regret that I could not have made it a more professional product.

- I played a useful role in the Metropolitan Washington Public Health Association and the Reconstructionist Havurah.

In my personal and family life—

- I tried to help Shirley overcome the depression that was rooted in her troubled childhood. I tried to make her happy. I believe we achieved a measure of success.

- We raised three children whom I love and of whom I am proud.

- We gained three grandchildren whom we saw grow from birth to maturity, and whom I love.

- In my retirement years I have found Marilyn, a new love and a new companion.

- Social relationships were not my strong suit. Casual conversations were not my forte.
- Economically we rose from uncertainty about which bill to pay, to a comfortable balance and a secure retirement.

What, then, is my legacy? What do I leave behind?

Three children who carry on the Seeman tradition of service to community. And their children, who will have their Seeman children.

Community service agencies that I founded and that serve needs today and onward.

And sincere, heart-warming, and productive relationships with friends, and work colleagues.

I sometimes reflect on the people whose lives I have touched, directly or indirectly. They are innumerable. Some very close, some unknown. With those I knew, I have made it a firm principle: honesty, integrity, sincerity, friendship. To my family. To the many volunteers who gave service to the community through the agencies I managed. To my associates at work. To those I will never know who are served by the agencies I helped create.

And now this autobiography.

Autobiography appears to be a Seeman tradition. My mother wrote a brief one. Will wrote a psychobiography as a project in graduate school. Shirley wrote a biography, and Mef wrote of his wonderful life with Alice. And now mine.

For Marilyn—

We Have Each Other
How fortunate we are to have each other.

We are two together,
Who belong together,
Each fulfilling the other.

We are a pair,
Who need to share,
And share we do.

Each gives to the other,
And each takes the best.
Together we fulfill.

Each alone is diminished;
Together we flourish.
We must believe it was meant to be.

How fortunate we are to have each other
In love.

CELEBRATING 99
2014

Marilyn had a great idea about how to celebrate my 99th birthday. At Riderwood there is a thriving Riderwood Jewish Community that holds erev Shabbat services in the Chapel every other week. After the service there is an oneg Shabbat, a dessert table with challah, wine, grape juice and a sweet table. The oneg is sponsored by members to memorialize or celebrate occasions.

She reserved the service nearest my birthday and sponsored the oneg in my honor. I was called up for an aleya, the reciting of the blessing before and after the reading of the week's Torah portion. All three of my sons had a part in the service: David opened the Ark, Jonathan said the blessing over the Challah, and Philip said the blessing over the wine. Jamie also joined the family on the bimah.

Many friends surrounded me during the oneg with warm congratulations. It was a happy affair.

A Change at 99
2014

Many of my friends and many other people I encounter regularly comment that I do not look as old as 99. I was active and independent and mobile. But 99 did catch up with me.

I had known that I had mild anemia for some time, but in the fall of 2014 I was diagnosed with serious anemia. There was also a concern that there might be internal bleeding related to the anemia. I was hospitalized and given several blood transfusions. They also performed an endoscopy. It turned out that they found no abnormalities in the upper gastro-intestinal system. At the same time I developed sciatica. A more severe pain I could not imagine; just miserable, even with pain medication. In time the sciatica cleared itself up. After a few days, I was transferred from the hospital to the rehabilitation unit at Riderwood.

At the rehab unit they discovered that I had picked up an infectious diarrhea at the hospital, a serious condition. *C.difficile colitis*. I returned to the hospital for treatment of the infection. After a few days, I returned to Riderwood rehab. It was surprising and troubling to learn how debilitating it is to spend so many days in a hospital, flat on your bed, hardly ever leaving the bed. The muscles atrophy.

At the rehab unit I spent 35 days with physical and occupational therapy daily, with excellent therapists. They taught me to use the walker. Marilyn visited every day, usually having a meal with me in the dining room. I now am confined to using a walker.

As for the Rest....
2016

For the last 26 years the focus of my professional work has been the study of mortality. It is no surprise, then, that at 99 I contemplate my own death. I do not fear death, neither do I welcome it. With ample time to reflect, I think I am prepared. I know well, that, as Shakespeare had Claudius, the usurping King of Denmark, say to console Hamlet, grieving over his father's death at the King's hand, "All that live must die."

I know that I, Isadore Seeman, as all other beings, have one pass on this earth, and then become an anonymous part of it for eternity. Nature decrees it. It is not a pleasant knowledge, but it is so.

CPSIA information can be obtained at www.ICGtesting.com
Printed in the USA
BVOW11s2240120116

432572BV00005B/7/P

9 780961 451936